Chiropractic Assistant

\-

The Comprehensive Guide

by

VIRUTI SHIVAN

Masters in Clinical Psychology (Major)

"In books, as in life, it's not the size or looks but the content that matters."

DISCLAIMER: The information in this book is provided for general informational purposes only and is not intended as professional advice. Although every effort has been made to ensure the accuracy and completeness of the information, the author and publisher do not assume responsibility for errors, inaccuracies, omissions, inconsistencies, or the impact of future advancements or updates in technology and information. This book is not a substitute for proper training, diagnosis, treatment, or guidance from qualified professionals. Readers are encouraged to consult experts in the relevant fields and independently verify the information when necessary. Any slights of people, places, or organizations are unintentional and purely coincidental.

Introduction

Welcome to "Chiropractic Assistant - The Comprehensive Guide," a resource designed to serve as your navigator through the intricate and rewarding landscape of chiropractic care. This guide is the culmination of years of experience, research, and a deep understanding of the chiropractic field, tailored to empower chiropractic assistants at all stages of their career. From those taking their first steps into the clinic to seasoned veterans looking to refine their skills and knowledge, this book aims to be an invaluable companion.

Chiropractic care is a unique and vital component of the healthcare system, focusing on the diagnosis, treatment, and prevention of mechanical disorders of the musculoskeletal system, especially the spine. As a chiropractic assistant, you play a crucial role in the smooth operation of the chiropractic clinic, the effective care of patients, and the overall success of the practice. Your responsibilities span a wide range, including patient care, administrative tasks, and clinic management. This guide will walk you through each of these areas, offering insights, strategies, and practical advice to enhance your performance and contribution.

The role of a chiropractic assistant is as challenging as it is rewarding, requiring a blend of interpersonal skills, technical know-how, and a compassionate approach to patient care. Through this guide, you will explore the foundational principles of chiropractic care, advanced knowledge on various chiropractic practices, and the nuances of patient communication and education. You will also delve into the operational aspects of clinic management, from office administration to optimizing health clinic workflows and integrating technology into your practice.

This book is structured to provide a comprehensive learning experience. Each chapter is divided into four subchapters, concluding with an exercise section containing 10 multiple-choice questions (MCQs) to test your understanding of the material. The absence of images or illustrations is a deliberate choice to focus on in-depth explanations and storytelling, bringing concepts to life through personal anecdotes and hypothetical scenarios. These narratives are designed to enrich your learning experience, making complex ideas more relatable and easier to grasp.

As we embark on this journey together, remember that your role as a chiropractic assistant is pivotal to the healing and well-being of countless individuals. Your dedication, knowledge, and care can transform lives, providing both physical relief and emotional support to those in need. Let this guide be your roadmap to excellence in the chiropractic field, as you continue to grow, learn, and make a significant impact on the health and lives of your patients.

Welcome to the beginning of an enriching journey toward becoming an indispensable part of the chiropractic community.

Chapter 1: The Role of a Chiropractic Assistant

1.1 Understanding Your Impact in the Chiropractic Field

The Foundation of Chiropractic Support

The role of a chiropractic assistant extends far beyond the day-to-day administrative tasks and patient management. You are the backbone of the chiropractic office, facilitating a smooth operation that allows chiropractors to focus on patient care. Your role is pivotal in creating a healing environment for patients, often being the first point of contact and the last smile they see as they leave. Understanding your impact on both the clinic's workflow and patient experience is crucial for personal and professional fulfillment in this role.

Bridging Communication Gaps

Effective communication is a cornerstone of any healthcare setting, and as a chiropractic assistant, you are often the translator between the chiropractor's medical jargon and the patient's understanding. Your ability to convey treatment plans, care instructions, and wellness advice in a clear and empathetic manner can significantly enhance patient compliance and satisfaction. This connection not only improves health outcomes but also fosters a trusting relationship between the patient and the clinic.

Enhancing Patient Experience

The chiropractic assistant's touchpoint extends to the ambiance of the clinic and the overall patient journey. From the moment a patient walks into the clinic, your role in managing appointments, ensuring comfort in the waiting area, and preparing them for their session contributes to their overall experience. This holistic approach to patient care often results in higher patient retention rates and positive word-of-mouth referrals, which are invaluable to the clinic's reputation and success.

Supporting Clinical Excellence

Behind every successful chiropractor, there is an efficient chiropractic assistant ensuring that the clinic operates like a well-oiled machine. Your responsibilities may include managing patient records, ensuring compliance with healthcare regulations, and keeping the clinic stocked with necessary supplies. By maintaining an organized and efficient workflow, you enable chiropractors to maximize their time with patients, thereby enhancing the quality of care delivered.

Personal and Professional Growth

The dynamic nature of the chiropractic field offers endless opportunities for learning and growth. By immersing yourself in the nuances of chiropractic care, you not only become more proficient in your role but also gain a deeper appreciation for the holistic approach to health. This knowledge empowers you to play a more active role in patient education and advocacy, further solidifying your position as an indispensable member of the healthcare team.

Conclusion

The role of a chiropractic assistant is multifaceted and deeply impactful. You are not just an administrative worker; you are a key player in the patient's healthcare journey, a facilitator of clinic efficiency, and a promoter of holistic well-being. Embracing the full scope of your impact in the chiropractic field is the first step toward achieving excellence and fulfillment in this rewarding career.

1.2 Skills Every Chiropractic Assistant Must Develop

Effective Communication

At the heart of a chiropractic assistant's skill set is effective communication. The ability to clearly convey information, listen attentively, and empathize with patients cannot be overstated. Whether it's explaining complex chiropractic procedures in simple terms or addressing patient concerns with sensitivity, your communication skills are vital in fostering a positive and reassuring clinic environment.

Organizational Prowess

Chiropractic assistants must excel in organizing not just the physical space of the clinic but also its operations. This includes managing patient appointments, keeping accurate and confidential patient records, and ensuring that supplies are well-stocked and equipment is maintained. An organized clinic runs smoothly, reduces stress for both staff and patients, and contributes to overall efficiency and productivity.

Adaptability and Problem-Solving

The healthcare environment is fast-paced and ever-changing. Chiropractic assistants must be adaptable, able to handle unexpected situations with grace, and find solutions to problems quickly. Whether it's dealing with a last-minute schedule change or resolving a patient issue, your ability to think on your feet is crucial in maintaining the flow of the clinic.

Technical Proficiency

In today's digital age, a chiropractic assistant must be proficient with various types of software, including electronic health records (EHR) systems, scheduling programs, and office productivity software. Understanding these tools not only improves the efficiency of your work but also ensures accuracy and compliance with healthcare regulations.

Patient Care and Empathy

A compassionate approach to patient care is essential. Chiropractic assistants often interact with patients who are in pain or discomfort. Showing empathy, understanding, and providing a comforting presence can make a significant difference in their experience and recovery. Your ability to demonstrate genuine care and concern is a powerful tool in creating a healing environment.

Team Collaboration

Working harmoniously within a team is a critical skill for chiropractic assistants. The ability to collaborate with chiropractors, other healthcare providers, and administrative staff ensures that the clinic operates seamlessly. Effective teamwork enhances the quality of patient care, promotes a positive work environment, and leads to better outcomes for everyone involved.

Attention to Detail

Finally, attention to detail is a non-negotiable skill for chiropractic assistants. From accurately inputting patient data to ensuring compliance with health and safety protocols, the smallest details can have significant implications. A meticulous approach to your work ensures high standards of care and operational excellence.

Developing these skills sets the foundation for a successful career as a chiropractic assistant. Beyond just fulfilling your responsibilities, these competencies allow you to contribute meaningfully to the wellbeing of patients and the efficiency of the clinic, making you an invaluable asset to any chiropractic team.

1.3 Navigating Patient Interactions with Compassion and Efficiency

Building a Foundation of Trust

Trust is the cornerstone of any patient-caregiver relationship. As a chiropractic assistant, your initial interactions set the tone for the patient's entire experience. Greet each patient warmly, make eye contact, and use their name to create a personal connection. Demonstrating active listening, acknowledging their concerns without interruption, and responding with empathy can significantly reinforce their trust in the care they are receiving.

Efficiency with a Human Touch

Efficiency does not have to come at the expense of compassion. Even in a busy clinic setting, strive to manage time effectively while ensuring each patient feels heard and valued. Implementing streamlined check-in procedures, maintaining a well-organized schedule, and being prepared for each patient's visit can help minimize wait times and reduce stress for both patients and staff.

Communicating Clearly and Concisely

Clear communication is vital in healthcare settings. When explaining appointments, procedures, or care instructions, use language that is easy to understand and avoid medical jargon. Encourage questions and provide answers that reassure and inform. Remember, a well-informed patient is more likely to be engaged in their care and follow through with treatment plans.

Handling Sensitive Situations

Chiropractic assistants often encounter patients experiencing pain, fear, or frustration. In such situations, maintaining professionalism while expressing genuine concern is key. Offer a listening ear, validate their feelings, and if a solution is within your capability, take swift action. If not, assure them you will escalate the matter to someone who can help. Handling sensitive situations with grace and tact strengthens the patient's confidence in the clinic.

Privacy and Confidentiality

Respect for patient privacy and confidentiality is non-negotiable. Be mindful of where and how you discuss patient information, ensuring conversations cannot be overheard by others not involved in their care. Adhering to privacy laws and clinic policies not only protects the patient but also builds their trust in your professionalism and the clinic's integrity.

Empowering Patients

Empowerment is a powerful aspect of patient care. Encourage patients to be active participants in their health and recovery. This can be achieved by providing educational materials, guiding them to resources, or simply offering encouragement and support for their efforts to follow through with treatment recommendations.

Follow-Up and Continuity of Care

Continuity of care is crucial for patient outcomes and satisfaction. Efficient follow-up procedures, whether for appointment reminders, checking on a patient's progress post-treatment, or managing ongoing care plans, demonstrate your commitment to their health and wellbeing. These interactions are opportunities to reinforce the patient's value to the clinic, encourage their continued engagement in their care, and address any emerging concerns.

Navigating patient interactions with compassion and efficiency requires a balance of soft skills and operational savvy. By fostering a supportive and understanding environment while ensuring the smooth functioning of clinic processes, chiropractic assistants play a pivotal role in enhancing patient experiences and outcomes.

1.4 Exercise: 10 MCQs with Answers at the End

1. What is the primary role of a chiropractic assistant in a clinic?

   A) Providing chiropractic adjustments

   B) Managing patient records and appointments

   C) Conducting initial patient assessments

   D) Prescribing medication

2. Effective communication for a chiropractic assistant includes:

A) Using complex medical terminology

B) Listening attentively and responding empathetically

C) Speaking quickly to save time

D) Avoiding eye contact to maintain professionalism

3. Which of the following is NOT a responsibility of a chiropractic assistant?

A) Diagnosing patient conditions

B) Ensuring the clinic is well-stocked with necessary supplies

C) Maintaining confidentiality of patient records

D) Scheduling patient appointments

4. Organizational skills in a chiropractic office include managing:

A) Only patient appointments

B) Only financial records

C) Patient appointments, records, and clinic supplies

D) The chiropractor's personal schedule

5. A chiropractic assistant shows empathy by:

A) Telling patients their feelings are unwarranted

B) Listening to and validating patient concerns

C) Rushing a patient through their appointment

D) Keeping conversations strictly professional

6. Team collaboration in a chiropractic clinic involves:

A) Working independently at all times

B) Sharing patient information without consent

C) Coordinating care with chiropractors and other staff

D) Avoiding communication with other healthcare providers

7. Which of the following best describes adaptability for a chiropractic assistant?

A) Unwillingness to learn new software programs

B) Inflexibility in handling unexpected schedule changes

C) Ability to handle unexpected situations with grace

D) Refusal to take on new responsibilities

8. Maintaining patient privacy and confidentiality is achieved by:

A) Discussing patient details in common areas

B) Sharing interesting patient cases on social media

C) Ensuring conversations about patients are private

D) Using patient names loudly in waiting areas

9. Empowering patients involves:

   A) Discouraging questions about their treatment plan

   B) Providing educational materials and resources

   C) Telling patients to follow instructions without explanation

   D) Ignoring patient feedback and concerns

10. Follow-up and continuity of care demonstrate:

   A) A lack of trust in the patient's ability to manage their health

   B) An unnecessary use of clinic resources

   C) Commitment to the patient's health and wellbeing

   D) The clinic's desire to charge patients more

Answers:

1. B) Managing patient records and appointments

2. B) Listening attentively and responding empathetically

3. A) Diagnosing patient conditions

4. C) Patient appointments, records, and clinic supplies

5. B) Listening to and validating patient concerns

6. C) Coordinating care with chiropractors and other staff

7. C) Ability to handle unexpected situations with grace

8. C) Ensuring conversations about patients are private

9. B) Providing educational materials and resources

10. C) Commitment to the patient's health and wellbeing

Chapter 2: Chiropractic Office Administration

2.1 Essentials of Clinic Management

Overview of Clinic Management

Effective clinic management is the linchpin of a successful chiropractic practice. It encompasses a wide range of responsibilities that ensure the clinic operates smoothly, efficiently, and provides high-quality patient care. At the heart of these operations is the chiropractic assistant, who plays a crucial role in managing day-to-day activities, from patient scheduling and record-keeping to financial management and compliance with healthcare regulations.

Patient Scheduling and Flow

One of the first pillars of clinic management is the efficient scheduling of patient appointments. This not only maximizes the chiropractor's time but also ensures patients are seen promptly and receive the attention they need without unnecessary delays. Effective scheduling strategies, such as considering the time needed for different types of appointments and allowing for buffer times, can significantly improve patient flow and satisfaction.

Record Keeping and Data Management

Accurate and confidential patient records are essential for providing high-quality care. These records include patient histories, treatment plans, and progress notes. Implementing a reliable electronic health record (EHR) system can streamline this process, making it easier to update and retrieve patient information. Additionally, proper data management practices ensure compliance with privacy laws and help safeguard sensitive patient information.

Financial Management

Financial health is critical to the clinic's longevity. This includes managing billing processes, insurance claims, and patient payments. A chiropractic assistant with a strong grasp of financial management can help optimize revenue cycles, reduce billing errors, and ensure that the clinic is compensated for the services provided. Furthermore, effective financial planning and budgeting are necessary to control costs and allocate resources efficiently.

Compliance and Legal Requirements

Navigating the complex landscape of healthcare regulations is another crucial aspect of clinic management. Staying informed about changes in healthcare laws, insurance policies, and professional standards is necessary to maintain compliance and avoid legal pitfalls. Regular training and updates for all clinic staff on these regulations can help prevent violations that could result in fines or damage to the clinic's reputation.

Quality Control and Improvement

Continuous improvement in patient care and clinic operations should be a constant goal. This involves regularly assessing and refining treatment protocols, patient satisfaction, and operational efficiency. Implementing quality control measures, such as patient feedback surveys and staff performance evaluations, can identify areas for improvement and drive the clinic towards excellence.

Professional Development and Staff Training

Investing in the professional development of staff, including chiropractic assistants, is essential for maintaining a high standard of care. Ongoing training and education ensure that the team is knowledgeable about the latest chiropractic practices, technologies, and management strategies. A well-trained team can provide better patient care, improve clinic operations, and adapt to the evolving healthcare landscape.

Conclusion

The essentials of clinic management form the foundation of a thriving chiropractic practice. By mastering these core areas, chiropractic assistants can significantly contribute to the clinic's success. Effective management not only enhances patient care and satisfaction but also ensures the clinic's operational efficiency and financial stability. In this dynamic role, chiropractic assistants are pivotal in navigating the challenges and opportunities within the healthcare industry, steering their clinics toward a prosperous future.

2.2 Record Keeping and Confidentiality

The Backbone of Patient Care

Record keeping is a fundamental aspect of chiropractic office administration, serving as the backbone of patient care and clinic integrity. Accurate, detailed, and timely records support the provision of high-quality chiropractic care by chronicling patient histories, treatments, and outcomes. These records facilitate effective communication among care providers and ensure continuity of care for patients.

Ensuring Accuracy and Timeliness

The chiropractic assistant is often responsible for the entry and updating of patient records. This task requires a meticulous attention to detail to ensure the accuracy of patient information, treatment notes, and billing data. Timeliness is also crucial; records must be updated promptly to reflect the most current information, which is vital for making informed treatment decisions and for legal compliance.

Confidentiality: A Legal and Ethical Obligation

Confidentiality is paramount in healthcare settings. Chiropractic assistants must understand and adhere to laws and regulations governing patient privacy, such as the Health Insurance Portability and Accountability Act (HIPAA) in the United States. This includes safeguarding patient information from unauthorized access, discussing patient information only with authorized individuals, and ensuring that physical and electronic records are securely stored.

Electronic Health Records (EHRs)

The adoption of Electronic Health Records (EHRs) has transformed record-keeping practices. EHRs offer numerous advantages over traditional paper records, including improved accessibility, reduced risk of errors, and enhanced security features. Chiropractic assistants should be proficient in using EHR systems, understanding their functionalities for recording, retrieving, and managing patient information.

Best Practices for Record Management

Effective record management involves more than just entering data into a system. It includes:

- Regular audits of records to ensure accuracy and completeness.

- Training on privacy laws and clinic policies for all staff members.

- Implementation of secure access controls and data encryption for electronic records.

- Development of protocols for responding to data breaches or unauthorized access incidents.

Patient Rights and Access to Records

Patients have the right to access their health records, and chiropractic assistants play a key role in facilitating this process.

It is important to handle such requests with professionalism, ensuring that patients receive the information they need in a timely manner, while also verifying the identity of the requester to protect patient privacy.

Ethical Considerations

Ethical considerations in record keeping and confidentiality extend beyond legal requirements. Respecting patient privacy fosters trust and supports the therapeutic relationship. It is essential to always act in the best interest of the patient, treating their information with the utmost respect and discretion.

Conclusion

Record keeping and confidentiality are critical components of chiropractic office administration, requiring a high level of professionalism, attention to detail, and ethical conduct. By adhering to best practices and legal standards, chiropractic assistants ensure the protection of patient information, contributing to the delivery of safe and effective chiropractic care.

2.3 Appointment Scheduling and Patient Flow

Optimizing Appointment Scheduling

Efficient appointment scheduling is a cornerstone of successful chiropractic office administration, directly impacting patient satisfaction and clinic productivity. A well-managed schedule minimizes wait times, maximizes the chiropractor's availability, and ensures a steady patient flow. To achieve this, chiropractic assistants must balance the clinic's capacity with patient demand, taking into account the varying lengths of appointments and the need for flexibility in case of emergencies or cancellations.

Strategies for Effective Scheduling

- **Buffer Times:** Incorporate buffer times between appointments to accommodate unforeseen delays and ensure each patient receives adequate time with the chiropractor.

- **Categorization of Appointment Types:** Differentiate appointment types (e.g., initial consultations, follow-up treatments, emergency visits) and allocate appropriate time slots for each to streamline scheduling.

- **Online Scheduling Tools:** Utilize online scheduling tools to allow patients to book appointments conveniently while enabling the clinic to manage its schedule efficiently.

- **Patient Reminders:** Implement a system for patient reminders via email, text, or phone calls to reduce no-shows and last-minute cancellations, thus maintaining a consistent patient flow.

Managing Patient Flow

Effective management of patient flow within the clinic is just as important as the scheduling of appointments. The goal is to ensure a smooth and timely transition of patients from their arrival through to the completion of their visit, enhancing their overall experience and minimizing congestion in the waiting area.

Key Elements of Managing Patient Flow:

- **Check-In Process:** Streamline the check-in process through digital check-in systems or efficient front-desk protocols to quickly move patients from arrival to the waiting area.

- **Waiting Area Management:** Maintain a comfortable and engaging waiting area, providing updates on wait times to manage patient expectations.

- **Treatment Room Turnover:** Ensure swift turnover of treatment rooms between appointments, keeping them clean and prepared for the next patient.

- **Post-Treatment Procedures:** Develop efficient post-treatment procedures, including check-out and future appointment scheduling, to keep the patient flow moving smoothly.

Leveraging Technology

Technology plays a vital role in optimizing both appointment scheduling and patient flow. Electronic scheduling systems can offer real-time visibility into the clinic's schedule, allowing for better decision-making and flexibility. Automated reminder systems help reduce no-shows, and digital check-in systems can streamline the arrival process, improving the overall efficiency of patient flow.

Communication and Flexibility

Open communication with patients about their appointments and wait times is crucial. Being upfront about delays can significantly improve patient satisfaction, as it shows respect for their time. Flexibility in handling emergencies, accommodating walk-ins, or rescheduling appointments also contributes to a positive patient experience and efficient clinic operations.

Conclusion

Appointment scheduling and patient flow are fundamental aspects of chiropractic office administration that require careful planning, effective use of technology, and clear communication. By adopting best practices in these areas, chiropractic assistants can significantly enhance clinic efficiency, patient satisfaction, and the overall success of the practice.

2.4 Exercise: 10 MCQs with Answers at the End

1. What is the primary goal of efficient appointment scheduling in a chiropractic clinic?

   A) Increase the workload on chiropractic assistants

   B) Minimize wait times and maximize chiropractor availability

   C) Discourage new patients from booking appointments

   D) Complicate the scheduling process

2. Buffer times between appointments are important because they:

A) Allow patients to leave the clinic later

B) Provide a margin for scheduling errors

C) Accommodate unforeseen delays and ensure adequate time for each patient

D) Decrease the number of appointments per day

3. Online scheduling tools benefit chiropractic clinics by:

A) Increasing paperwork

B) Allowing patients to book appointments at their convenience

C) Making it difficult for staff to manage appointments

D) Reducing patient satisfaction

4. Patient reminders are used to:

A) Increase no-shows

B) Reduce no-shows and last-minute cancellations

C) Confuse patients with their appointment times

D) Overwhelm patients with communication

5. Effective patient flow management aims to:

A) Increase waiting time for patients

B) Ensure a smooth transition of patients through their clinic visit

C) Create congestion in the waiting area

D) Discourage patients from completing post-treatment procedures

6. Streamlining the check-in process can be achieved through:

A) Longer forms for patients to fill out upon arrival

B) Digital check-in systems or efficient front-desk protocols

C) Ignoring patients as they arrive

D) Creating a complicated check-in procedure

7. The purpose of maintaining a comfortable and engaging waiting area is to:

A) Make the wait feel longer

B) Manage patient expectations regarding wait times

C) Discourage patients from staying

D) Increase patient anxiety

8. Technology enhances appointment scheduling and patient flow by:

A) Slowing down processes

B) Offering real-time visibility and decision-making flexibility

C) Increasing the likelihood of scheduling mistakes

D) Reducing clinic efficiency

9. Flexibility in appointment scheduling is crucial for:

A) Only prioritizing long-term patients

B) Handling emergencies and accommodating walk-ins

C) Making it difficult for new patients to get appointments

D) Decreasing the clinic's adaptability to patient needs

10. Open communication with patients about appointments and wait times:

A) Decreases patient satisfaction

B) Shows disrespect for their time

C) Is unnecessary in a professional setting

D) Improves patient satisfaction by respecting their time

Answers:

1. B) Minimize wait times and maximize chiropractor availability

2. C) Accommodate unforeseen delays and ensure adequate time for each patient

3. B) Allowing patients to book appointments at their convenience

4. B) Reduce no-shows and last-minute cancellations

5. B) Ensure a smooth transition of patients through their clinic visit

6. B) Digital check-in systems or efficient front-desk protocols

7. B) Manage patient expectations regarding wait times

8. B) Offering real-time visibility and decision-making flexibility

9. B) Handling emergencies and accommodating walk-ins

10. D) Improves patient satisfaction by respecting their time

Chapter 3: Basics of Chiropractic Care

3.1 The Philosophy Behind Chiropractic Medicine

Holistic Approach to Health

The philosophy of chiropractic medicine is grounded in the holistic approach to health, emphasizing the body's intrinsic ability to heal itself. This perspective considers not just the physical symptoms but the overall well-being of the patient, including mental, emotional, and lifestyle factors. Chiropractic care is based on the premise that proper alignment of the body's musculoskeletal structure, particularly the spine, will enable the body to heal itself without surgery or medication.

The Central Role of the Spine

At the heart of chiropractic philosophy is the belief that the spine is central to maintaining optimal health. The spine's health is crucial because it houses and protects the spinal cord, which is part of the central nervous system. The nervous system controls and coordinates all the body's functions, and any misalignment (subluxations) can affect the body's ability to function and heal. Chiropractors focus on correcting these subluxations to restore health and prevent disease.

Prevention and Maintenance

Another key aspect of chiropractic philosophy is the emphasis on prevention and maintenance of health rather than just the treatment of disease. Regular chiropractic adjustments are seen as a way to maintain the optimal function of the musculoskeletal and nervous systems, preventing potential health issues before they arise. This proactive approach to health encourages patients to take an active role in their wellness, incorporating healthy lifestyle choices and regular chiropractic care.

The Body as an Integrated System

Chiropractic medicine views the body as an integrated system, where every part is interconnected and affects the whole. This means that a problem in one area of the body could cause symptoms in another area. Chiropractors assess the entire body to identify the root cause of a patient's symptoms, rather than just treating the symptoms themselves. This comprehensive approach ensures that the underlying issues are addressed, promoting long-term health and well-being.

Patient Empowerment

Central to the chiropractic philosophy is the empowerment of patients to take charge of their health. Education on posture, ergonomics, nutrition, exercise, and stress management is often part of chiropractic care. By equipping patients with the knowledge and tools to maintain their health, chiropractors foster a partnership with patients in their journey towards optimal wellness.

Conclusion

The philosophy behind chiropractic medicine offers a unique and holistic approach to health and wellness, emphasizing the body's natural healing abilities, the importance of the spine and nervous system, and the value of preventative care. By understanding and embracing this philosophy, both chiropractors and patients can work together towards achieving and maintaining optimal health.

3.2 Common Chiropractic Treatments and Techniques

Spinal Manipulation and Adjustment

The cornerstone of chiropractic care, spinal manipulation and adjustment, involves the application of controlled force to spinal joints that are experiencing abnormal movement patterns or fail to function normally. The objective is to restore mobility, alleviate pain, and muscle tightness, and allow tissues to heal. Chiropractors use their hands or a small instrument to apply a sudden yet controlled force to a spinal joint, often resulting in an audible release of gas (a cracking or popping sound) that indicates improved joint mobility.

Mobilization Techniques

In contrast to the direct force used in spinal adjustments, mobilization techniques involve low-velocity movements and stretches of muscles and joints, with the goal of increasing the range of motion within those areas. This method is particularly beneficial for patients who require a gentler approach due to pain or specific conditions.

Soft Tissue Therapy

Chiropractors employ various soft tissue therapies to treat muscle, ligament, and tendon problems. Techniques such as myofascial release, trigger point therapy, and massage are used to release tension in the soft tissues, improve circulation, and reduce inflammation, thereby aiding in the healing process and pain relief.

Flexion-Distraction Technique

This gentle, non-force spinal manipulation is performed on a special table that moves as the chiropractor manipulates the spine. The flexion-distraction technique is mainly used to treat disc injuries with or without leg pain (sciatica). It increases spinal motion and resolves disc bulges and herniations, reducing pressure on the spinal nerves.

Instrument-Assisted Soft Tissue Mobilization (IASTM)

IASTM involves the use of specially designed instruments to gently massage and scrape the skin. This technique helps to break down scar tissue, fascial restrictions, and adhesions in the soft tissues, leading to improved range of motion and reduced pain.

Therapeutic Exercises and Stretches

Chiropractors often prescribe specific therapeutic exercises and stretches to patients to help maintain the results achieved through manual treatment. These exercises help strengthen the muscles, improve flexibility, and protect against new injuries or the recurrence of previous conditions.

Dietary and Nutritional Counseling

Recognizing the importance of diet and nutrition in overall health, chiropractors may offer advice and plans to help improve their patients' diet. Proper nutrition supports the body's healing processes and can complement chiropractic care in achieving optimal health.

Lifestyle Modification Counseling

Lifestyle changes can significantly impact one's health and well-being. Chiropractors often provide counseling on lifestyle modifications that can help reduce stress, improve sleep quality, and increase physical activity, thereby enhancing the effectiveness of chiropractic treatments.

Conclusion

Chiropractic care encompasses a wide array of treatments and techniques aimed at promoting optimal health and well-being. By addressing the root causes of pain and dysfunction through a holistic approach, chiropractors are able to offer their patients a path towards improved health without the need for invasive treatments or medications.

3.3 The Anatomy and Physiology in Chiropractic Care

Understanding the Spine's Structure

The spine is a complex anatomical structure that plays a central role in chiropractic care. It consists of 33 vertebrae, divided into five regions: cervical, thoracic, lumbar, sacrum, and coccyx. These vertebrae encase and protect the spinal cord while supporting the body's weight and allowing a wide range of motion. Intervertebral discs, situated between each vertebra, act as shock absorbers and provide flexibility to the spine. Understanding the spine's anatomy is crucial for chiropractors to diagnose issues and administer effective treatments.

The Nervous System's Role

Chiropractic care emphasizes the importance of the nervous system, which comprises the brain, spinal cord, and peripheral nerves. It controls and coordinates all bodily functions. Subluxations or misalignments in the spine can interfere with nerve signal transmission, leading to various health issues. By correcting these subluxations, chiropractic adjustments aim to restore optimal nervous system function and promote the body's natural healing abilities.

Musculoskeletal System Interactions

The musculoskeletal system includes bones, muscles, tendons, and ligaments that provide support, stability, and movement to the body. Chiropractic care addresses imbalances and dysfunctions in this system, focusing on how these issues can lead to pain, reduced mobility, and impaired health. Techniques such as adjustments, mobilization, and soft tissue therapy help to relieve tension, improve alignment, and enhance musculoskeletal function.

Biomechanics and Movement

Chiropractors have a deep understanding of biomechanics, or how the body moves. This knowledge allows them to identify abnormalities in gait, posture, and movement patterns that can contribute to pain and dysfunction. Corrective exercises and advice on proper posture and ergonomics are often part of chiropractic treatment plans, aimed at improving movement efficiency and preventing further injury.

The Role of Inflammation and Pain

Inflammation is a natural response of the body to injury or disease but can lead to pain and tissue damage if it becomes chronic. Chiropractic care seeks to reduce inflammation through techniques that restore proper joint function and support tissue healing. This approach not only alleviates pain but also addresses the underlying causes of inflammation, promoting long-term health.

Healing and Recovery Processes

Chiropractic treatments stimulate the body's healing mechanisms by improving blood flow, reducing nerve interference, and enhancing lymphatic drainage. This holistic approach supports the body's ability to heal itself from injuries, reduces reliance on medication for pain management, and prevents chronic conditions from developing.

Preventative Care and Wellness

Anatomy and physiology are not only pivotal in treating existing conditions but also in preventing future health problems. Chiropractors use their knowledge to educate patients on how to maintain optimal spinal health, engage in healthy lifestyle practices, and achieve balance and wellness in their lives.

Conclusion

The principles of anatomy and physiology are fundamental to chiropractic care, guiding the diagnosis and treatment of various conditions. By focusing on the intricate relationship between the body's structure and function, chiropractors provide a unique and effective approach to health care that promotes healing, restores function, and enhances overall well-being.

3.4 Exercise: 10 MCQs with Answers at the End

1. What is the primary focus of chiropractic care?

   A) Prescription medications

   B) Surgery

   C) Spinal adjustments and manipulation

D) Invasive procedures

2. How many vertebrae are there in a typical human spine?

A) 23

B) 33

C) 28

D) 30

3. What part of the nervous system is primarily involved in chiropractic treatments?

A) Peripheral nervous system

B) Central nervous system

C) Autonomic nervous system

D) Somatic nervous system

4. Which region of the spine contains the most vertebrae?

A) Cervical

B) Thoracic

C) Lumbar

D) Sacral

5. What is the role of intervertebral discs?

  A) To provide nutrients to the spine

  B) To act as shock absorbers

  C) To connect the spinal cord to the brain

  D) To limit the movement of the vertebrae

6. Chiropractic adjustments aim to correct what?

  A) Broken bones

  B) Subluxations

  C) Muscle tears

  D) Arterial blockages

7. The nervous system controls and coordinates all bodily functions through what?

  A) Blood circulation

  B) Hormonal release

  C) Nerve impulses

  D) Muscle contractions

8. What technique might a chiropractor use to treat soft tissue injuries?

  A) Ice pack application

  B) Myofascial release

C) Antibiotics

D) Blood transfusions

9. How can improper posture affect the body according to chiropractic philosophy?

   A) It has no significant effect

   B) It improves blood flow

   C) It can lead to subluxations and pain

   D) It increases cognitive function

10. What is a primary goal of preventative chiropractic care?

   A) To diagnose diseases

   B) To perform surgeries

   C) To maintain spinal health and prevent dysfunction

   D) To prescribe medications for chronic conditions

Answers:

1. C) Spinal adjustments and manipulation

2. B) 33

3. B) Central nervous system

4. B) Thoracic

5. B) To act as shock absorbers

6. B) Subluxations

7. C) Nerve impulses

8. B) Myofascial release

9. C) It can lead to subluxations and pain

10. C) To maintain spinal health and prevent dysfunction

Chapter 4: Advanced Chiropractic Knowledge

4.1 Understanding Complex Chiropractic Conditions

Introduction to Complex Conditions

In the realm of chiropractic care, practitioners often encounter complex conditions that require a deeper understanding of the body's intricacies. These conditions can challenge the conventional approach to treatment and necessitate a comprehensive, integrative strategy. Understanding these complex chiropractic conditions involves recognizing their multifaceted nature, underlying causes, and the potential for interdisciplinary care approaches.

Degenerative Disc Disease (DDD)

Degenerative Disc Disease is a condition characterized by the deterioration of one or more intervertebral discs, which can lead to chronic pain, reduced mobility, and other neurological symptoms. Despite its name, DDD is not a disease but a natural consequence of aging. Chiropractors approach DDD with techniques aimed at improving joint mobility, reducing pain, and enhancing the quality of life through spinal adjustments, physical therapy, and lifestyle recommendations.

Sciatica

Sciatica refers to pain that radiates along the path of the sciatic nerve, which extends from the lower back down through the legs. This condition is often caused by a herniated disc or bone spur pressing on the nerve. Chiropractic treatment for sciatica may include spinal adjustments, ice/cold therapy, and exercises designed to relieve nerve compression and pain.

Fibromyalgia

Fibromyalgia is a complex condition characterized by widespread musculoskeletal pain, fatigue, sleep, memory, and mood issues. While the exact cause of fibromyalgia is unknown, chiropractic care can play a significant role in managing symptoms. Techniques focus on improving sleep quality, reducing pain and stiffness, and enhancing overall well-being through a combination of adjustments, soft tissue therapies, and guidance on exercise and nutrition.

Scoliosis

Scoliosis involves an abnormal lateral curvature of the spine and can range from mild to severe. Chiropractic care for scoliosis aims to reduce discomfort, improve function, and prevent further progression of the curve. Treatment may include specific spinal adjustments, corrective exercises, and the use of supportive devices.

Whiplash and Other Auto Injury-Related Conditions

Whiplash is a common injury resulting from auto accidents, characterized by rapid forward and backward neck movement. This can lead to neck pain, stiffness, headaches, and other symptoms. Chiropractic treatment for whiplash focuses on restoring movement, reducing pain, and facilitating the healing process through spinal adjustments and muscle relaxation techniques.

Integrative Approaches to Care

For complex chiropractic conditions, an integrative approach that combines chiropractic care with other healthcare modalities can be highly effective. This may involve collaboration with medical doctors, physical therapists, and other specialists to provide a holistic treatment plan that addresses all aspects of the patient's health.

Educating Patients

Educating patients about their conditions, treatment options, and ways to prevent further issues is an essential part of managing complex chiropractic conditions. This empowers patients to take an active role in their healthcare and supports better long-term outcomes.

Conclusion

Understanding and treating complex chiropractic conditions requires a deep knowledge of the body's structure and functions, as well as a commitment to ongoing learning and collaboration with other healthcare professionals. By adopting a comprehensive and patient-centered approach, chiropractors can effectively manage these challenging conditions and significantly improve their patients' quality of life.

4.2 Innovations in Chiropractic Treatment

The field of chiropractic care is continuously evolving, with new technologies and methodologies enhancing the effectiveness of treatments and expanding the scope of conditions that can be managed. These innovations not only improve patient outcomes but also contribute to the broader acceptance and integration of chiropractic care within the healthcare system.

Laser Therapy

One of the most significant advancements in chiropractic treatment is the introduction of laser therapy, particularly Low-Level Laser Therapy (LLLT). LLLT uses specific wavelengths of light to interact with tissue and is known to accelerate the healing process by increasing circulation, reducing inflammation, and encouraging tissue repair. This non-invasive therapy is effective for a variety of conditions, including chronic pain, soft tissue injuries, and arthritis.

Spinal Decompression Therapy

Spinal decompression therapy is a modern, non-surgical technique aimed at relieving back pain and other problems associated with spinal disc injuries. Controlled, gentle spinal decompression machines stretch the spine, creating a vacuum that can help reposition bulging discs and draw necessary nutrients into the disc. This therapy is particularly beneficial for patients with herniated discs, sciatica, or degenerative disc disease.

Digital Posture Analysis

The development of digital posture analysis tools has revolutionized the way chiropractors assess and treat posture-related issues. These tools provide a detailed, accurate assessment of a patient's posture, highlighting imbalances and areas of stress that could lead to pain or dysfunction. This technology enables chiropractors to develop more targeted treatment plans and track progress over time.

Functional Movement Screening (FMS)

FMS is a screening tool that evaluates the quality of movement patterns to identify limitations and asymmetries which can reduce the effectiveness of functional movements and increase the risk of injury. By incorporating FMS into their practice, chiropractors can customize treatment and exercise programs to address specific movement deficiencies, improving overall physical performance and preventing injuries.

Nutrigenomics in Chiropractic Care

Nutrigenomics is an emerging field that examines the relationship between nutrition and genetic expression. Chiropractors who embrace this approach offer dietary and nutritional advice tailored to the individual's genetic makeup, enhancing the body's ability to heal and maintain optimal health. This personalized approach to nutrition represents a significant shift towards more holistic, integrative care strategies.

Instrument-Assisted Soft Tissue Mobilization (IASTM) Tools

Innovations in IASTM tools have enhanced the effectiveness of soft tissue therapy. Ergonomically designed instruments made from advanced materials allow chiropractors to more precisely target and treat soft tissue dysfunctions, promoting faster recovery and improved range of motion.

Virtual Reality (VR) for Rehabilitation

VR technology is beginning to make its way into chiropractic rehabilitation. By simulating real-life scenarios in a controlled environment, VR can help patients improve balance, coordination, and motor skills in a safe, engaging manner. This technology holds promise, especially for patients recovering from injuries or those with mobility issues.

Conclusion

These innovations in chiropractic treatment not only showcase the field's commitment to continuous improvement but also highlight its potential to provide more comprehensive, effective care. As research advances and technology evolves, chiropractic care will likely play an increasingly significant role in holistic health care and the management of a broad range of conditions.

4.3 Integrative Approaches to Chiropractic Care

Integrative approaches in chiropractic care represent a blending of traditional chiropractic techniques with a wide range of complementary therapies. This holistic perspective aims to treat the whole person, not just the symptoms, by addressing physical, emotional, nutritional, and lifestyle factors that contribute to well-being.

Collaboration with Other Healthcare Professionals

A key component of integrative chiropractic care is the collaboration with other healthcare professionals, such as physical therapists, acupuncturists, nutritionists, and medical doctors. This multidisciplinary approach ensures that patients receive a comprehensive treatment plan that addresses all aspects of their health, leading to more effective outcomes.

Physical Therapy and Rehabilitation

Incorporating physical therapy and rehabilitation exercises into chiropractic treatment plans enhances recovery by improving strength, flexibility, and endurance. These exercises are tailored to each patient's specific needs, helping to correct imbalances and prevent future injuries.

Acupuncture and Traditional Chinese Medicine (TCM)

Acupuncture, a key component of TCM, is increasingly used alongside chiropractic adjustments to provide pain relief, reduce inflammation, and promote healing. The combination of these practices can offer a powerful synergistic effect, improving patient outcomes, especially in cases of chronic pain and musculoskeletal conditions.

Nutritional Counseling and Supplementation

Nutrition plays a vital role in healing and overall health. Integrative chiropractic care often includes nutritional counseling and the use of supplements to support the body's natural healing processes, boost the immune system, and improve energy levels. Tailored dietary advice can also help manage inflammation, which is often a contributing factor to musculoskeletal pain.

Stress Management Techniques

Stress can significantly impact physical health, including exacerbating pain and hindering the healing process. Chiropractors employing an integrative approach may introduce stress management techniques such as meditation, yoga, and deep breathing exercises to help patients manage stress and improve their overall health and well-being.

Lifestyle Modifications

Guidance on lifestyle modifications is another important aspect of integrative chiropractic care. By addressing factors such as sleep quality, physical activity, and ergonomics, chiropractors help patients make changes that support their health and reduce the risk of injury or illness.

Functional Medicine

Functional medicine seeks to identify and address the root causes of diseases, looking at the body as an integrated system. Some chiropractors incorporate functional medicine principles into their practice, using detailed histories and advanced diagnostic testing to develop personalized treatment plans that can include diet, exercise, and detoxification programs.

Conclusion

Integrative approaches to chiropractic care represent a comprehensive strategy to health and wellness, combining the best of traditional chiropractic methods with a broad spectrum of complementary therapies. This holistic approach not only addresses specific health issues but also promotes overall well-being, enabling patients to achieve and maintain optimal health.

4.4 Exercise: 10 MCQs with Answers at the End

1. What is the main goal of integrative chiropractic care?

   A) To prescribe medications

   B) To perform surgeries

C) To treat symptoms only

D) To treat the whole person

2. Which professional might a chiropractor collaborate with in an integrative approach?

A) Nutritionist

B) Accountant

C) Electrician

D) Lawyer

3. What role does physical therapy play in integrative chiropractic care?

A) It is used to improve billing practices

B) It is unrelated to chiropractic care

C) It enhances recovery by improving physical function

D) It replaces the need for chiropractic adjustments

4. How does acupuncture complement chiropractic care in an integrative approach?

A) By providing legal advice

B) By improving energy flow and reducing pain

C) By decorating the clinic

D) By managing the clinic's finances

5. What is the purpose of including nutritional counseling in chiropractic care?

A) To increase the clinic's revenue

B) To improve the patient's dietary habits for better health outcomes

C) To teach cooking classes

D) To sell unnecessary supplements

6. Why are stress management techniques incorporated into chiropractic care?

A) To make the treatment sessions longer

B) Because they are trendy

C) To address the impact of stress on physical health

D) To distract patients from their symptoms

7. Which is NOT a focus of lifestyle modifications recommended by chiropractors?

A) Improving sleep quality

B) Increasing physical activity

C) Enhancing workplace ergonomics

D) Reducing educational pursuits

8. How does functional medicine complement chiropractic care?

A) By focusing on acute injuries only

B) By identifying and addressing the root causes of diseases

C) By ignoring lifestyle factors

D) By limiting the scope of treatment to spinal adjustments

9. What is a key component of the integrative approach in chiropractic care?

A) Isolation from other healthcare fields

B) Collaboration with other healthcare professionals

C) Avoidance of any physical therapy techniques

D) Sole focus on chiropractic adjustments without additional therapies

10. Which statement best describes the integrative approach to chiropractic care?

A) It prioritizes medication over natural healing processes

B) It considers only the physical symptoms presented by the patient

C) It integrates a variety of complementary therapies and lifestyle changes

D) It rejects the use of modern technology in treatments

Answers:

1. D) To treat the whole person

2. A) Nutritionist

3. C) It enhances recovery by improving physical function

4. B) By improving energy flow and reducing pain

5. B) To improve the patient's dietary habits for better health outcomes

6. C) To address the impact of stress on physical health

7. D) Reducing educational pursuits

8. B) By identifying and addressing the root causes of diseases

9. B) Collaboration with other healthcare professionals

10. C) It integrates a variety of complementary therapies and lifestyle changes

Chapter 5: Patient Communication and Education

5.1 Effective Communication Techniques

Effective communication is vital in building a trusting relationship between chiropractors (and chiropractic assistants) and their patients. It not only enhances patient satisfaction but also improves treatment outcomes by ensuring patients fully understand their diagnosis, treatment options, and the importance of follow-up care.

Active Listening

Active listening involves giving full attention to the speaker, understanding their message, responding thoughtfully, and remembering the information. It allows chiropractic professionals to understand patient concerns and symptoms better, making patients feel valued and respected.

Empathy

Empathy is the ability to understand and share the feelings of another. Expressing empathy towards patients can significantly impact their comfort and trust level, making them more likely to share important health information and adhere to treatment plans.

Clear and Simple Language

Using clear and simple language free of medical jargon is crucial when communicating with patients. It ensures that patients understand their condition and the proposed treatment, empowering them to make informed decisions about their health care.

Patient Education

Educating patients about their condition and the benefits of chiropractic care is an integral part of effective communication. Providing resources, such as brochures or links to reputable websites, can further enhance their understanding and engagement with their treatment plan.

Visual Aids

Visual aids, including anatomical models and diagrams, can help patients visualize their condition and how treatments work. They are especially useful in explaining complex concepts or procedures.

Open-ended Questions

Asking open-ended questions encourages patients to express their concerns and symptoms in detail. This not only provides chiropractors with a better understanding of the patient's condition but also promotes a dialogue that can lead to more personalized care.

Feedback and Confirmation

Seeking feedback and confirmation ensures that the patient has understood the information provided. Asking patients to summarize what they have learned or to ask questions about any unclear areas can help identify and address any misunderstandings promptly.

Cultural Competence

Being culturally competent means understanding and respecting the diverse backgrounds of patients, including their beliefs, values, and customs. This awareness can significantly enhance communication and patient care by ensuring that treatment plans are sensitive to and respectful of cultural differences.

Follow-up Communication

Follow-up communication, whether through phone calls, emails, or text messages, shows patients that their care team is invested in their recovery and well-being. It also provides an opportunity to address any questions or concerns that may arise after an appointment.

Conclusion

Effective communication is a cornerstone of successful chiropractic care. By implementing these techniques, chiropractic professionals can foster a positive and healing environment that encourages patient engagement, improves compliance with treatment plans, and ultimately leads to better health outcomes.

5.2 Educating Patients on Chiropractic Care

Educating patients about chiropractic care is essential not only for enhancing their understanding of the treatment but also for empowering them to take an active role in their health and wellness journey. This education process can demystify chiropractic practices, reduce anxieties, and build a foundation of trust and cooperation between patients and chiropractic professionals.

Introduction to Chiropractic Principles

Start by introducing patients to the basic principles of chiropractic care, emphasizing the body's innate ability to heal itself and the central role of the spine and nervous system in overall health. Explain how chiropractic adjustments work to restore proper alignment and nerve function, thereby improving health outcomes.

Benefits of Chiropractic Care

Highlight the benefits of chiropractic care, including pain relief, improved mobility, enhanced nervous system function, and better quality of life. Use evidence-based research to support these claims, helping patients understand the value and effectiveness of chiropractic treatments.

Common Conditions Treated

Inform patients about the common conditions that chiropractic care can treat, such as back pain, neck pain, headaches, and musculoskeletal issues. This can help patients relate their own symptoms to the potential benefits of chiropractic adjustments, encouraging them to pursue treatment.

What to Expect During a Chiropractic Session

Describe what patients can expect during their first and subsequent chiropractic sessions. Include information on the initial consultation, examination, diagnosis, and treatment plan. Clarify any misconceptions about the safety and discomfort of chiropractic adjustments to alleviate fears and set realistic expectations.

The Role of Patients in Their Care

Emphasize the importance of patient participation in their care. Discuss the role of lifestyle choices, exercise, and ergonomics in supporting chiropractic treatments. Encourage patients to ask questions and express their concerns, fostering a collaborative approach to health care.

Long-term Health and Preventative Care

Educate patients on the role of chiropractic care in long-term health and wellness, including preventative care. Highlight how regular chiropractic adjustments, coupled with a healthy lifestyle, can prevent future issues and maintain optimal health.

Resources for Further Education

Provide patients with resources for further education, such as brochures, reputable websites, and recommended readings. Directing patients to reliable sources can prevent misinformation and further solidify their understanding and trust in chiropractic care.

Success Stories and Testimonials

Sharing success stories and testimonials from other patients can be a powerful tool in patient education. These stories can inspire confidence in the efficacy of chiropractic care and demonstrate its impact on improving patients' quality of life.

Conclusion

Educating patients on chiropractic care is a crucial component of the treatment process. By providing clear, comprehensive information, chiropractic professionals can demystify treatment procedures, underscore the benefits of care, and engage patients in a partnership aimed at achieving the best possible health outcomes.

5.3 Handling Sensitive Conversations

Sensitive conversations are an integral part of patient care in chiropractic practice, requiring a delicate balance of professionalism, empathy, and clear communication. Whether discussing a challenging diagnosis, addressing treatment anxieties, or navigating through patient frustrations, the approach to these conversations can significantly impact patient trust and treatment outcomes.

Establish a Comfortable Environment

Begin by ensuring the conversation takes place in a private, quiet setting where the patient feels secure and respected. A comfortable environment fosters openness, allowing patients to express their concerns without fear of judgment.

Use Empathetic Listening

Empathy is at the core of handling sensitive conversations. Listen attentively to the patient's concerns, validating their feelings and acknowledging their experiences. This approach demonstrates care and understanding, laying the groundwork for a constructive dialogue.

Communicate Clearly and Compassionately

When conveying information that might be difficult for the patient to hear, do so with both clarity and compassion. Avoid medical jargon, and ensure the patient fully understands the situation. Be direct yet gentle, offering support and reassurance throughout the conversation.

Provide Support and Options

Patients facing challenging situations need to feel supported and not alone. Offer them a range of options whenever possible, and discuss the next steps in their care or treatment. Empowering patients with choices can help alleviate feelings of helplessness or despair.

Maintain Professionalism

While empathy and understanding are essential, maintaining professionalism is equally important. Ensure that the conversation remains focused on the patient's care and well-being, steering clear of personal opinions or non-evidence-based recommendations.

Invite Questions

Encourage patients to ask questions, and provide clear, honest answers. Addressing their concerns directly can help reduce anxiety and build trust. If you don't have an immediate answer, commit to finding it and follow up promptly.

Offer Additional Resources

For patients needing more support, recommend additional resources such as support groups, counseling services, or educational materials. These resources can provide further assistance and information, helping patients navigate through their concerns more effectively.

Document the Conversation

Make a note of the conversation in the patient's records, including any concerns raised and the information provided. Documentation ensures continuity of care and helps inform future discussions.

Follow Up

Sensitive conversations shouldn't end when the patient leaves the room. Follow up with the patient to check on their well-being, answer new questions that may have arisen, and offer ongoing support. This continued care reinforces the patient's value and your commitment to their health.

Conclusion

Handling sensitive conversations with care, empathy, and professionalism is a critical skill in chiropractic practice. By adopting these techniques, chiropractors and chiropractic assistants can ensure these discussions are productive and supportive, enhancing patient trust and fostering a positive therapeutic relationship.

5.4 Exercise: 10 MCQs with Answers at the End

1. What is a key component of effective communication in chiropractic care?

   A) Ignoring patient concerns

   B) Using complex medical terminology

   C) Active listening

   D) Speaking quickly

2. Empathy in patient communication is important for:

   A) Decreasing treatment time

   B) Increasing clinic revenue

   C) Building trust and understanding

   D) Simplifying medical procedures

3. Clear and simple language helps to:

   A) Confuse patients

   B) Ensure patients understand their condition and treatment

   C) Make conversations quicker

   D) Avoid detailed explanations

4. Educating patients about chiropractic care is crucial for:

   A) Making patients dependent on the chiropractor

   B) Empowering patients to take an active role in their health

   C) Limiting patient questions

   D) Discouraging self-care practices

5. Visual aids in patient education can:

   A) Complicate the learning process

   B) Help patients visualize their condition and treatment

   C) Decrease patient satisfaction

   D) Increase treatment costs unnecessarily

6. Open-ended questions encourage:

   A) Short, uninformative responses

   B) Detailed patient responses

   C) Patients to leave quickly

   D) Misunderstandings

7. Handling sensitive conversations with empathy and professionalism can:

   A) Undermine patient confidence

   B) Build trust and strengthen the patient-practitioner relationship

C) Discourage patients from sharing their concerns

D) Make patients feel unwelcome

8. Providing support and options to patients during sensitive conversations:

A) Limits patient autonomy

B) Makes patients feel overwhelmed

C) Helps alleviate feelings of helplessness

D) Reduces the effectiveness of treatment

9. Encouraging patients to ask questions and providing clear answers:

A) Wastes time during appointments

B) Can help reduce patient anxiety

C) Is unnecessary for informed consent

D) Decreases patient trust

10. Follow-up after sensitive conversations is important for:

A) Checking on the patient's well-being and offering ongoing support

B) Increasing the number of appointments

C) Avoiding further communication

D) Reducing clinic liability

Answers:

1. C) Active listening

2. C) Building trust and understanding

3. B) Ensure patients understand their condition and treatment

4. B) Empowering patients to take an active role in their health

5. B) Help patients visualize their condition and treatment

6. B) Detailed patient responses

7. B) Build trust and strengthen the patient-practitioner relationship

8. C) Helps alleviate feelings of helplessness

9. B) Can help reduce patient anxiety

10. A) Checking on the patient's well-being and offering ongoing support

Chapter 6: Health Clinic Workflow Optimization

6.1 Streamlining Daily Operations

Optimizing the workflow within a chiropractic clinic is essential for enhancing patient care, improving staff efficiency, and increasing overall clinic productivity. Streamlining daily operations involves evaluating and refining processes to reduce waste, eliminate unnecessary steps, and ensure that resources are utilized effectively.

Implementing Electronic Health Records (EHR)

One of the most significant steps toward streamlining operations is the adoption of Electronic Health Records (EHR). EHR systems facilitate quick access to patient records, streamline the documentation process, and improve communication among healthcare providers. They also support appointment scheduling, billing, and reporting functions, making them indispensable tools for efficient clinic management.

Automating Appointment Scheduling and Reminders

Utilizing online scheduling tools allows patients to book their appointments at their convenience, reducing the workload on front-desk staff. Automated appointment reminders, sent via

SMS or email, can significantly reduce no-show rates, ensuring a smoother flow of patients throughout the day.

Optimizing Patient Check-in and Check-out Processes

Streamlining the check-in and check-out processes can significantly enhance patient experience and clinic efficiency. Implementing digital check-in systems, such as tablets or kiosks, enables patients to fill out forms electronically, saving time and reducing paperwork. Similarly, a streamlined check-out process, with clear instructions for follow-up care and easy payment options, ensures a positive end to the patient's visit.

Standardizing Procedures and Protocols

Developing and implementing standard operating procedures (SOPs) for common tasks and treatments ensures consistency and efficiency. SOPs help new staff members quickly learn the clinic's processes and allow for the delegation of tasks without compromising the quality of care.

Regular Training and Staff Development

Investing in regular training and development for all staff members enhances their skills and knowledge, leading to improved patient care and operational efficiency. Training sessions can cover a range of topics, from customer service best practices to the latest advancements in chiropractic care.

Effective Inventory Management

An efficient inventory management system ensures that the clinic always has the necessary supplies without overstocking. Regularly reviewing inventory levels, setting reorder points, and leveraging inventory management software can help maintain optimal stock levels and prevent disruptions in care.

Leveraging Data for Continuous Improvement

Collecting and analyzing data on various aspects of clinic operations, from patient satisfaction to appointment wait times, provides valuable insights that can drive continuous improvement. Identifying bottlenecks and areas for improvement helps to streamline workflows and enhance the overall efficiency of the clinic.

Conclusion

Streamlining daily operations in a chiropractic clinic not only improves the work environment for staff but also enhances the patient experience. By embracing technology, standardizing processes, and fostering a culture of continuous improvement, chiropractic clinics can achieve a level of operational efficiency that supports high-quality care and contributes to the clinic's success.

6.2 Implementing Efficient Systems and Processes

Efficiency in a chiropractic clinic goes beyond mere organization; it's about creating a system that maximizes productivity and enhances patient care. Implementing efficient systems and processes is crucial for maintaining a smooth operation that can adapt to the growing needs of the clinic and its patients.

Patient Flow Management

Optimizing patient flow is essential to minimize wait times and ensure a comfortable and satisfactory experience. This involves careful scheduling to avoid overbooking, designing the clinic layout to reduce bottlenecks, and clearly marking different areas such as reception, waiting rooms, treatment rooms, and checkout to facilitate easy movement.

EHR and Practice Management Software

Investing in comprehensive Electronic Health Records (EHR) and practice management software streamlines administrative tasks, from scheduling appointments to billing and coding. These systems can also offer insights into practice trends, helping to make informed decisions about resource allocation and services offered.

Digital Communication Platforms

Leveraging digital communication platforms enhances the connection between the clinic and its patients. Secure messaging, online appointment booking, and telehealth services can improve access to care, reduce administrative burdens, and keep patients engaged in their health management.

Task Automation

Automating routine tasks can significantly improve clinic efficiency. This includes appointment reminders, patient follow-ups, and inventory alerts. Automation reduces the risk of human error and frees up staff time for more patient-centered activities.

Cross-training Staff

Cross-training staff members ensure that the clinic can operate smoothly even in the absence of key personnel. It enables staff to perform multiple roles, increasing flexibility in scheduling and ensuring that patient care is not compromised.

Quality Improvement Initiatives

Continuous quality improvement initiatives are vital for identifying inefficiencies and implementing solutions. Regular staff meetings to discuss challenges and opportunities for improvement can foster a culture of innovation and teamwork.

Streamlined Billing and Coding Processes

Efficient billing and coding processes are crucial for financial sustainability. This includes accurate documentation, timely submission of claims, and effective management of denials and appeals. Training staff on the latest billing codes and insurance requirements can reduce errors and delays in payment.

Feedback Mechanisms

Establishing mechanisms for receiving and acting on feedback from both patients and staff is critical for continuous improvement. Surveys, suggestion boxes, and regular review sessions can provide valuable insights into areas needing enhancement.

Conclusion

Implementing efficient systems and processes in a chiropractic clinic is a dynamic and ongoing effort that requires commitment from all staff members. By focusing on areas such as patient flow, digitalization, automation, and quality improvement, clinics can achieve operational excellence, leading to better patient outcomes, higher staff satisfaction, and overall clinic success.

6.3 Enhancing Patient Experience through Workflow Management

Enhancing the patient experience is a critical goal for any chiropractic clinic, directly impacting patient satisfaction, retention, and the overall success of the practice. Effective workflow management plays a pivotal role in achieving this by ensuring that every aspect of the patient's journey, from arrival to follow-up, is smooth, efficient, and centered around their needs.

Streamlined Check-in Process

The patient experience begins the moment they enter the clinic. A streamlined check-in process, facilitated by digital tools such as online pre-appointment forms and electronic check-in kiosks, can significantly reduce wait times and administrative burdens. Ensuring that this process is quick and hassle-free sets a positive tone for the entire visit.

Comfortable Waiting Areas

While minimizing wait times is ideal, ensuring that any necessary waiting periods are comfortable and stress-free is also crucial. Comfortable seating, a calm atmosphere, and access to water, reading materials, or even Wi-Fi can make the waiting area a positive space for patients.

Effective Communication During the Visit

Clear and compassionate communication throughout the patient's visit is essential. This includes explaining procedures, answering questions, and providing guidance on what to expect next. Ensuring that patients feel heard, understood, and cared for enhances their experience and trust in the clinic.

Efficient Treatment Rooms

The layout and organization of treatment rooms should facilitate efficient care while also making patients feel comfortable and safe. Essential supplies should be readily accessible to reduce treatment time and ensure that the chiropractor can focus entirely on the patient.

Personalized Patient Care

Tailoring the care experience to meet individual patient needs is fundamental to enhancing their experience. This can include personalized treatment plans, consideration of patient preferences, and accommodating special requests whenever possible. Recognizing and treating patients as individuals can significantly impact their satisfaction and loyalty.

Follow-up and Ongoing Engagement

The patient experience extends beyond their time in the clinic. Effective follow-up communication, whether for care instructions, appointment reminders, or check-ins on the patient's progress, demonstrates ongoing commitment to their health. Additionally, providing educational resources and wellness tips can keep patients engaged and motivated in their health journey.

Leveraging Technology for Convenience

Technology, such as patient portals and mobile apps, can offer patients convenient access to their health information, appointment scheduling, and direct communication with their chiropractor. These tools enhance the patient experience by empowering them with control over their health care.

Soliciting and Acting on Feedback

Regularly soliciting feedback from patients about their experience and making tangible improvements based on this feedback shows that the clinic values their input and is committed to continuous improvement. This not only enhances patient satisfaction but can also lead to better clinic practices and patient outcomes.

Conclusion

Managing workflows with a focus on enhancing patient experience is a strategic approach that benefits both patients and the clinic. By streamlining processes, emphasizing communication, personalizing care, and leveraging technology, chiropractic clinics can create a patient-centered environment that fosters satisfaction, loyalty, and positive health outcomes.

6.4 Exercise: 10 MCQs with Answers at the End

1. What is the primary goal of workflow management in a chiropractic clinic?

  A) To increase paperwork

  B) To enhance patient experience

  C) To limit patient interaction

  D) To reduce staff numbers

2. Which feature can significantly improve the check-in process for patients?

  A) Lengthy paper forms

  B) Digital pre-appointment forms

  C) Complicated procedures

  D) Manual record-keeping

3. What contributes to a comfortable waiting area?

  A) Uncomfortable seating

  B) Limited space

  C) Access to amenities like water and Wi-Fi

  D) Loud noises

4. Effective communication during a patient's visit is crucial for:

A) Confusing the patient

B) Enhancing patient experience

C) Increasing treatment time

D) Reducing interaction

5. The layout and organization of treatment rooms should:

A) Be cluttered

B) Facilitate efficient care

C) Limit access to essential supplies

D) Make the chiropractor's job harder

6. Personalized patient care includes:

A) Ignoring patient preferences

B) One-size-fits-all treatment plans

C) Tailoring treatment to individual needs

D) Avoiding special requests

7. Effective follow-up communication demonstrates:

A) A lack of professional boundaries

B) An ongoing commitment to patient health

C) Disinterest in patient feedback

D) The clinic's desire to overcharge

8. Leveraging technology for convenience can provide patients with:

A) Less control over their health care

B) Confusing medical information

C) Access to their health information and appointment scheduling

D) Unreliable health advice

9. Soliciting and acting on feedback shows:

A) The clinic values patient input

B) The clinic is indecisive

C) Patient opinions are unimportant

D) Feedback is a formality without real purpose

10. Streamlining daily operations in a chiropractic clinic aims to:

A) Complicate patient care

B) Reduce the quality of service

C) Improve efficiency and patient satisfaction

D) Increase patient wait times

Answers:

1. B) To enhance patient experience

2. B) Digital pre-appointment forms

3. C) Access to amenities like water and Wi-Fi

4. B) Enhancing patient experience

5. B) Facilitate efficient care

6. C) Tailoring treatment to individual needs

7. B) An ongoing commitment to patient health

8. C) Access to their health information and appointment scheduling

9. A) The clinic values patient input

10. C) Improve efficiency and patient satisfaction

Chapter 7: Ethical Considerations in Chiropractic Practice

7.1 Navigating Ethical Dilemmas

Ethical dilemmas in chiropractic practice often arise when there are conflicting values, beliefs, or principles at play. These situations can challenge chiropractors to make decisions that uphold the integrity of their profession while ensuring the best outcomes for their patients. Navigating these dilemmas requires a deep understanding of ethical principles and a commitment to professional standards.

Understanding Ethical Principles

Key ethical principles in healthcare include autonomy, beneficence, non-maleficence, and justice. Autonomy respects the patient's right to make informed decisions about their care. Beneficence involves acting in the best interest of the patient, while non-maleficence means doing no harm. Justice refers to treating all patients fairly and without discrimination. Chiropractors must balance these principles when facing ethical dilemmas.

Common Ethical Dilemmas in Chiropractic Care

- **Informed Consent:** Ensuring patients fully understand their treatment options, the risks and benefits, and alternative therapies.

- **Professional Boundaries:** Maintaining a professional relationship with patients, avoiding conflicts of interest, and managing dual relationships.

- **Confidentiality:** Protecting patient privacy and information, especially in small communities or when using digital records.

- **Overutilization of Services:** Addressing the ethical concerns related to unnecessary treatments or prolonging therapy beyond the patient's needs.

Strategies for Navigating Ethical Dilemmas

- **Ethical Decision-Making Models:** Utilize established models for ethical decision-making that guide through a structured process, considering all relevant factors and outcomes.

- **Continuing Education:** Engage in ongoing education on ethical issues and professional standards to stay informed about best practices and emerging concerns.

- **Consultation and Collaboration:** Seek advice from colleagues, professional associations, or ethics committees when faced with complex ethical decisions.

- **Transparent Communication:** Maintain open and honest communication with patients, providing clear information and listening to their concerns and preferences.

- **Documentation:** Keep thorough records of decisions made and the rationale behind them, especially when deviating from standard practices.

Creating an Ethical Practice Environment

Building an ethical practice environment is foundational to navigating ethical dilemmas. This involves:

- **Setting Clear Policies:** Develop and enforce policies on confidentiality, informed consent, professional boundaries, and ethical billing practices.

- **Fostering an Ethical Culture:** Encourage a practice culture where ethical considerations are openly discussed, and staff are empowered to raise concerns.

- **Lead by Example:** Practice leaders should exemplify ethical behavior, demonstrating commitment to professional standards and patient care.

Conclusion

Navigating ethical dilemmas in chiropractic practice demands a principled approach, rooted in a deep understanding of ethical principles and a commitment to upholding the highest standards of patient care. By employing strategies such as ethical decision-making models, continuous education, and creating an ethical practice environment, chiropractors can effectively manage these challenges, ensuring their practice not only complies with professional ethics but also serves the best interests of their patients.

7.2 Confidentiality and Patient Rights

Confidentiality and the protection of patient rights are paramount in chiropractic practice, as in all healthcare settings. These principles are critical for maintaining trust between patients and healthcare providers, ensuring the privacy and dignity of individuals seeking care.

Understanding Confidentiality

Confidentiality involves safeguarding personal information shared by patients during the course of their care. This includes medical history, treatment plans, and any personal details disclosed in the healthcare setting. Breaches of confidentiality can erode patient trust, harm the patient-provider relationship, and lead to legal consequences.

Legal and Ethical Obligations

Chiropractors, like all healthcare providers, are bound by legal and ethical obligations to protect patient confidentiality. Laws such as the Health Insurance Portability and Accountability Act (HIPAA) in the United States set standards for the handling and sharing of health information. Adherence to these laws is not just a legal requirement but a moral imperative to respect patient privacy.

Patient Rights

Patients have rights regarding their healthcare information, including the right to access their medical records, request corrections, and be informed about how their information is used and shared. Chiropractors must ensure patients are aware of these rights and facilitate their exercise without undue barriers.

Challenges to Confidentiality

Challenges to maintaining confidentiality can arise in various scenarios, such as discussions in open areas, electronic record-keeping, and interactions with third parties like insurance companies. Implementing strict privacy policies, using secure communication channels, and ensuring staff are trained in confidentiality practices are essential measures to mitigate these risks.

Informed Consent and Privacy

Informed consent is closely linked to confidentiality, as patients must be informed about how their information will be used and shared as part of their care. Clear communication about privacy practices and obtaining explicit consent for the use of patient information are crucial steps in respecting patient autonomy and rights.

Handling Breaches of Confidentiality

In the event of a breach of confidentiality, it is important to act swiftly to address the issue, inform affected patients, and take steps to prevent future breaches. This includes reviewing and strengthening privacy policies and practices, as well as providing additional training for staff.

Ethical Considerations in Information Sharing

Ethical considerations come into play when sharing patient information for purposes such as referrals, research, or public health reporting. Even in these contexts, the principle of minimum necessary information applies, and patient consent should be sought whenever possible.

Conclusion

Confidentiality and the protection of patient rights are foundational to ethical and effective chiropractic practice. By upholding these principles, chiropractors not only comply with legal requirements but also build a foundation of trust and respect with their patients, contributing to the overall quality and effectiveness of care.

7.3 The Importance of Professional Conduct

Professional conduct within chiropractic care encompasses a wide range of behaviors and practices that are critical to maintaining the trust and respect of patients, colleagues, and the community. It involves adhering to ethical standards, demonstrating competence and integrity, and committing to continuous improvement and patient-centered care.

Upholding Ethical Standards

The cornerstone of professional conduct is a steadfast commitment to ethical standards. Chiropractors are expected to practice with honesty, integrity, and fairness, treating all patients with respect and dignity. Ethical practice also means prioritizing patient welfare, avoiding conflicts of interest, and maintaining confidentiality.

Demonstrating Competence and Care

Competence in chiropractic practice is not just about technical skill but also about communication, decision-making, and patient care. Demonstrating competence involves staying informed about the latest research and advancements in the field, applying evidence-based practices, and tailoring treatments to meet the unique needs of each patient.

Integrity and Accountability

Integrity in professional conduct means doing the right thing, even when it's not the easiest option. It involves being accountable for one's actions, admitting mistakes, and taking corrective action when necessary. Chiropractors must ensure that their practice is transparent, and they should be willing to undergo scrutiny to uphold the highest standards of care.

Professional Development and Lifelong Learning

The healthcare field, including chiropractic care, is continually evolving. Commitment to professional development and lifelong learning is essential for staying current with best practices, emerging technologies, and new research findings. This commitment not only enhances the quality of care provided to patients but also contributes to the advancement of the chiropractic profession.

Collaboration and Respect in the Healthcare Community

Professional conduct extends to interactions with other healthcare providers. Collaborating with other professionals, referring patients when appropriate, and engaging in interdisciplinary care teams are practices that emphasize the chiropractor's role in the broader healthcare ecosystem. Mutual respect and collaboration can lead to more comprehensive care for patients and a more integrated approach to health and wellness.

Patient-Centered Care and Communication

At the heart of professional conduct is a commitment to patient-centered care. This involves listening to patients, respecting their preferences and values, and involving them in decision-making processes. Effective communication, empathy, and a genuine concern for patient well-being are essential aspects of professional conduct that can significantly impact patient satisfaction and treatment outcomes.

Community Engagement and Public Education

Professional conduct also involves engaging with the community and contributing to public education about chiropractic care, health, and wellness. By participating in community events, offering workshops, and providing resources, chiropractors can enhance public understanding of chiropractic care and its role in maintaining and improving health.

Conclusion

The importance of professional conduct in chiropractic practice cannot be overstated. It is foundational to building trust, ensuring quality care, and fostering a positive reputation for the profession. By adhering to ethical standards, demonstrating competence, and committing to continuous improvement and patient-centered care, chiropractors can significantly impact the health and well-being of their patients and the community.

7.4 Exercise: 10 MCQs with Answers at the End

1. What is the foundation of professional conduct in chiropractic practice?

   A) Financial gain

   B) Ethical standards

   C) Minimal patient interaction

   D) Competition with other healthcare providers

2. Professional competence in chiropractic care includes:

A) Ignoring new research and developments

B) Prioritizing personal beliefs over patient care

C) Staying informed about the latest advancements in the field

D) Avoiding collaboration with other healthcare professionals

3. Integrity in professional conduct means:

A) Only admitting mistakes when caught

B) Doing the right thing, even when it's not the easiest option

C) Prioritizing the chiropractor's needs over the patient's

D) Keeping successful treatment methods secret

4. Continuous professional development is important for:

A) Maintaining the status quo

B) Enhancing the quality of care and contributing to the profession's advancement

C) Avoiding patient feedback

D) Reducing the need for patient consent

5. Collaboration with other healthcare providers demonstrates:

A) A lack of confidence in chiropractic care

B) The chiropractor's role in the broader healthcare ecosystem

C) Unwillingness to take responsibility for patient care

D) A preference for traditional medicine over chiropractic methods

6. Patient-centered care in chiropractic practice involves:

A) Disregarding patient preferences and values

B) Listening to patients and involving them in decision-making

C) Limiting information given to patients to prevent confusion

D) Encouraging dependence on chiropractic treatments

7. Community engagement and public education about chiropractic care:

A) Detracts from time spent with patients

B) Is irrelevant to professional conduct

C) Enhances public understanding and contributes to health and wellness

D) Should only be done for marketing purposes

8. Accountability in professional conduct requires:

A) Blaming others for mistakes

B) Transparency and willingness to undergo scrutiny

C) Keeping treatment errors secret

D) Avoiding feedback from peers and patients

9. Ethical dilemmas in chiropractic practice are best navigated through:

A) Avoidance and denial

B) Ethical decision-making models and consultation

C) Personal intuition without consulting others

D) Strict adherence to personal profit motives

10. The ultimate goal of upholding professional conduct in chiropractic care is to:

A) Increase clinic revenue at all costs

B) Build trust, ensure quality care, and foster a positive reputation

C) Minimize patient interactions and streamline clinic operations

D) Focus solely on the chiropractor's professional development

Answers:

1. B) Ethical standards

2. C) Staying informed about the latest advancements in the field

3. B) Doing the right thing, even when it's not the easiest option

4. B) Enhancing the quality of care and contributing to the profession's advancement

5. B) The chiropractor's role in the broader healthcare ecosystem

6. B) Listening to patients and involving them in decision-making

7. C) Enhances public understanding and contributes to health and wellness

8. B) Transparency and willingness to undergo scrutiny

9. B) Ethical decision-making models and consultation

10. B) Build trust, ensure quality care, and foster a positive reputation

Chapter 8: Professional Development for Chiropractic Assistants

8.1 Continuing Education and Certification

In the dynamic field of chiropractic care, the role of chiropractic assistants is crucial for the smooth operation of a clinic and the delivery of quality patient care. Continuing education and certification are key components of professional development for chiropractic assistants, enabling them to stay current with the latest practices, enhance their skills, and contribute more effectively to patient care and clinic operations.

Importance of Continuing Education

Continuing education is vital for chiropractic assistants to keep abreast of the evolving healthcare landscape, including new technologies, patient care techniques, and administrative practices. It ensures that they can adapt to changes and meet the needs of both the chiropractors they support and the patients they serve. Continuing education can also open up new opportunities for career advancement and specialization within the field.

Types of Continuing Education

Continuing education for chiropractic assistants can take many forms, including:

- **Workshops and Seminars:** These can cover a wide range of topics, from patient communication and office management to specific healthcare compliance issues and emerging chiropractic research.

- **Online Courses:** Many reputable institutions and professional organizations offer online courses designed specifically for chiropractic assistants, allowing for flexible learning schedules.

- **Conferences:** Attending professional conferences not only provides educational opportunities but also allows chiropractic assistants to network with peers and learn from leaders in the field.

Certification Programs

Certification for chiropractic assistants is a testament to their professionalism, competence, and dedication to their role. While requirements vary by location and institution, obtaining certification often involves completing an accredited program and passing an examination. Certification can enhance a chiropractic assistant's credentials and may be required by some employers.

Benefits of Certification

- **Recognition of Professionalism:** Certification demonstrates a commitment to maintaining high standards of care and professionalism.

- **Improved Patient Care:** Certified chiropractic assistants are equipped with the knowledge and skills to contribute more effectively to patient care and clinic success.

- **Career Advancement:** Certification can lead to better job prospects, higher salaries, and opportunities for advancement within the chiropractic field.

Maintaining Certification

Maintaining certification typically requires the completion of continuing education credits on a regular basis. This requirement encourages continuous learning and ensures that chiropractic assistants remain knowledgeable about the latest developments in their field.

Conclusion

Continuing education and certification are essential for the professional development of chiropractic assistants. By pursuing these opportunities, chiropractic assistants can enhance their skills, contribute more effectively to their clinics, and ensure the highest quality of patient care. Investing in professional development not only benefits the individual assistant but also strengthens the chiropractic profession as a whole.

8.2 Building a Career Path in Chiropractic Care

Embarking on a career within the realm of chiropractic care offers numerous pathways for growth, specialization, and personal fulfillment. Whether one begins as an assistant or a licensed practitioner, the journey involves continuous learning, skill enhancement, and adaptation to the evolving landscape of health and wellness.

Starting with a Strong Foundation

A solid educational background forms the cornerstone of a successful career in this field. For those aiming to advance from assistant roles to more clinical positions, obtaining a degree from an accredited institution is crucial. This foundational step ensures a deep understanding of human anatomy, physiology, and the principles of chiropractic methods.

Gaining Experience and Specialization

Hands-on experience is invaluable. Working closely with experienced practitioners provides practical insights into patient care, clinic operations, and the nuances of effective treatment strategies. Over time, individuals may find areas within chiropractic care that resonate deeply with their interests and skills. Specializing in areas such as sports injuries, pediatric care, or rehabilitation can differentiate one's practice and cater to specific patient needs.

Leveraging Continuing Education

The field of chiropractic care, like all healthcare professions, is subject to continuous scientific and technological advancements. Engaging in continuing education through workshops, seminars, and courses not only fulfills licensure requirements but also enriches one's knowledge base, keeping practitioners at the forefront of the field.

Professional Certification and Advancement

Obtaining additional certifications in specialized techniques or therapies can significantly enhance a practitioner's skill set and marketability. These certifications often require a combination of coursework and practical examinations, demonstrating a commitment to excellence and patient care.

Networking and Professional Associations

Building relationships with other professionals through networking events and memberships in professional associations can open doors to new opportunities. These connections provide support, mentorship, and insights into emerging trends, legislative changes, and practice management strategies.

Research and Contribution to the Field

Contributing to chiropractic research or engaging in scholarly activities can further one's career and the profession as a whole. Publishing findings, speaking at conferences, or teaching can establish an individual as a thought leader in the field.

Exploring Practice Ownership or Management

For those with an entrepreneurial spirit, opening a private practice or taking on managerial roles within existing clinics offers a pathway to professional autonomy and leadership. This step requires not only clinical expertise but also skills in business management, marketing, and human resources.

Conclusion

Building a career in chiropractic care is a dynamic process that involves lifelong learning, personal development, and a commitment to improving the health and well-being of patients. By embracing opportunities for education, specialization, and professional engagement, individuals can forge rewarding careers that make a significant impact on the lives of those they serve.

8.3 Networking and Professional Growth

Networking and professional growth are key components in the career development of individuals in the chiropractic field. Building connections and engaging in continuous learning can open up new opportunities, provide insights into the latest industry trends, and enhance one's skills and knowledge.

The Value of Professional Networking

Creating a network of peers, mentors, and industry experts is invaluable for anyone looking to advance their career in chiropractic care. Networking can lead to new job opportunities, collaborative projects, or partnerships that can enhance one's practice. It provides a platform for sharing experiences, challenges, and solutions, fostering a sense of community and support among professionals.

Ways to Network in the Chiropractic Field

- **Attend Industry Conferences and Workshops:** These events are excellent opportunities to meet other professionals, learn about the latest research and techniques, and engage with thought leaders in the field.

- **Join Professional Associations:** Membership in professional associations offers access to exclusive resources, educational materials, and networking events. It also signals a commitment to professional standards and continuing education.

- **Participate in Online Forums and Social Media Groups:** Online communities bring together chiropractic professionals from around the world, allowing for the exchange of ideas, advice, and experiences without geographical limitations.

- **Volunteer for Professional Committees or Boards:** Serving on committees or boards related to chiropractic care or healthcare in general can broaden one's network and contribute to the profession's advancement.

Benefits of Professional Growth

Engaging in activities that promote professional growth, such as obtaining additional certifications, attending advanced training sessions, or pursuing further education, can significantly enhance one's expertise and service offerings. This not only improves patient care but also increases the marketability and competitiveness of one's practice.

Mentorship

Both seeking mentorship and serving as a mentor can be powerful tools for professional development. Mentorship relationships provide guidance, support, and insight based on the mentor's experience, helping mentees navigate their career paths and overcome obstacles more effectively.

Contributing to the Profession

Contributing to the chiropractic community through research, writing articles, giving presentations, or teaching can establish an individual as a knowledgeable and respected professional. These contributions not only aid in personal growth but also help advance the field by disseminating new knowledge and best practices.

Lifelong Learning

The commitment to lifelong learning ensures that chiropractic professionals remain at the cutting edge of their field. Keeping abreast of new research, technologies, and treatment methodologies enables practitioners to offer the best possible care to their patients and maintain a thriving practice.

Conclusion

Networking and professional growth are essential for anyone in the chiropractic field looking to advance their career, enhance their practice, and contribute to the health and wellness of their community. Through active engagement with peers, continuous learning, and participation in the broader professional community, chiropractic professionals can achieve personal and professional fulfillment.

8.4 Exercise: 10 MCQs with Answers at the End

1. What is a primary benefit of networking in the chiropractic field?

    A) Increasing patient wait times

    B) Reducing the need for continuing education

    C) Opening up new job opportunities

    D) Decreasing clinic revenue

2. Which event is an effective way to meet other chiropractic professionals?

    A) Casual coffee meetings only

    B) Industry conferences and workshops

C) Solitary online research

D) Avoiding professional associations

3. Membership in professional associations can provide:

   A) Limited access to industry information

   B) Exclusive resources and educational materials

   C) A decrease in professional credibility

   D) An excuse to avoid networking

4. Online forums and social media groups offer:

   A) Geographical limitations to networking

   B) Opportunities for global professional exchange

   C) Few benefits to professional development

   D) An increased risk of malpractice

5. Additional certifications can:

   A) Decrease a practitioner's marketability

   B) Enhance expertise and service offerings

   C) Oversaturate a practice with unnecessary skills

   D) Limit professional growth opportunities

6. The role of a mentor in chiropractic care includes:

   A) Providing minimal guidance and support

   B) Offering insights based on experience

   C) Encouraging reliance on outdated practices

   D) Discouraging participation in professional development

7. Contributing to the chiropractic profession can be done through:

   A) Isolating oneself from the community

   B) Ignoring new research and developments

   C) Research, writing articles, and giving presentations

   D) Avoiding sharing knowledge with peers

8. Lifelong learning ensures chiropractic professionals:

   A) Fall behind in industry advancements

   B) Remain at the cutting edge of their field

   C) Lose interest in professional development

   D) Become overwhelmed by new information

9. Volunteering for professional committees or boards can:

   A) Broaden one's professional network

   B) Diminish the value of one's practice

   C) Limit exposure to new ideas

D) Reduce the quality of patient care

10. Attending advanced training sessions is beneficial for:

    A) Keeping practice methods outdated

    B) Improving patient care and competitiveness

    C) Decreasing professional standards

    D) Isolating a practice from industry trends

Answers:

1. C) Opening up new job opportunities

2. B) Industry conferences and workshops

3. B) Exclusive resources and educational materials

4. B) Opportunities for global professional exchange

5. B) Enhance expertise and service offerings

6. B) Offering insights based on experience

7. C) Research, writing articles, and giving presentations

8. B) Remain at the cutting edge of their field

9. A) Broaden one's professional network

10. B) Improving patient care and competitiveness

Chapter 9: Integrating Technology in Chiropractic Practice

9.1 The Role of Electronic Health Records (EHR)

The integration of technology in chiropractic practice, particularly through the use of Electronic Health Records (EHR), represents a significant advancement in healthcare management. EHR systems offer a comprehensive and streamlined approach to managing patient information, improving the quality of care, enhancing patient safety, and optimizing clinic operations.

Centralization of Patient Information

EHR systems centralize patient information, including medical history, treatment plans, diagnostic tests, and billing details, in one digital platform. This centralization facilitates easy access to patient data, enabling chiropractors and healthcare staff to make informed decisions quickly and efficiently.

Improved Quality of Care

With EHRs, healthcare providers can track patient progress over time, monitor treatment effectiveness, and adjust care plans as needed. The ability to access a patient's complete health record instantly supports a more coordinated and personalized approach to patient care.

Enhanced Patient Safety

EHRs contribute to patient safety by reducing the risk of errors associated with manual record-keeping and prescription management. Alerts and reminders within EHR systems can help prevent potential drug interactions, ensure timely follow-ups, and prompt critical health screenings, contributing to overall patient safety.

Streamlined Administrative Processes

EHR systems streamline administrative tasks such as appointment scheduling, billing, and insurance claims processing. Automated features reduce the time and effort required for these tasks, allowing chiropractic staff to focus more on patient care and less on paperwork.

Facilitating Compliance with Health Regulations

EHR systems are designed to help practices comply with healthcare regulations and standards, including privacy laws and documentation requirements. They offer secure storage and transmission of patient data, ensuring that patient information is protected according to legal guidelines.

Support for Telehealth Services

The role of EHRs extends to supporting telehealth services, which have become increasingly important in providing care to patients who cannot physically visit the clinic. EHR systems can facilitate virtual consultations, remote monitoring, and digital communication between patients and chiropractors, expanding access to chiropractic care.

Data Analytics and Quality Improvement

EHR systems often include data analytics capabilities, allowing practices to analyze trends, measure performance outcomes, and identify areas for improvement. This data can inform quality improvement initiatives, helping chiropractic practices enhance service delivery and patient satisfaction.

Patient Engagement and Education

EHRs can also play a role in patient engagement and education by providing patients with access to their health records, educational materials, and health management tools. This empowers patients to take an active role in their healthcare, leading to better health outcomes and increased patient satisfaction.

Conclusion

The role of Electronic Health Records in chiropractic practice is transformative, offering numerous benefits that extend beyond mere record-keeping. By improving the quality of care, enhancing patient safety, and streamlining administrative processes, EHRs support the delivery of efficient, effective, and patient-centered chiropractic care.

9.2 Utilizing Chiropractic Software

In the evolving landscape of chiropractic care, the utilization of specialized chiropractic software has become a game-changer. This technology is designed to meet the unique needs of chiropractic practices, streamlining operations, enhancing patient care, and improving overall practice management.

Practice Management Solutions

Chiropractic software often encompasses comprehensive practice management solutions, which include appointment scheduling, billing, and patient communication tools. These features simplify daily administrative tasks, allowing for more efficient clinic operations and more time spent on patient care.

Electronic Health Records (EHR) Integration

Many chiropractic software platforms offer seamless integration with Electronic Health Records (EHR), enabling a unified approach to patient information management. This integration ensures that patient records are easily accessible, up-to-date, and securely stored, facilitating better-informed treatment decisions and continuity of care.

Patient Engagement Tools

Patient engagement is crucial for successful treatment outcomes. Chiropractic software often includes patient portals, which provide patients with direct access to their health records, appointment scheduling, and secure messaging with their chiropractor. These tools empower patients to take an active role in their healthcare journey, improving communication and satisfaction.

Clinical Documentation and Reporting

Chiropractic software simplifies the process of clinical documentation, offering templates and customizable forms that make it easy to record patient encounters, treatment plans, and progress notes. Advanced reporting features allow for the analysis of practice trends, patient outcomes, and financial performance, supporting informed decision-making and strategic planning.

Billing and Insurance Processing

Efficient billing and insurance processing are vital for the financial health of any chiropractic practice. Chiropractic software streamlines these processes with automated billing, coding suggestions, and electronic claim submissions. This not only reduces administrative burdens but also helps to minimize errors and accelerate reimbursement.

Telehealth Capabilities

As telehealth becomes an increasingly important component of healthcare, chiropractic software that supports virtual consultations can extend the reach of chiropractic care. These capabilities allow chiropractors to provide services to patients who are unable to visit the clinic in person, ensuring continuity of care and expanding access to chiropractic services.

Customizable Treatment Plans

Software designed for chiropractic care often includes features for creating and managing customizable treatment plans. This functionality supports a personalized approach to patient care, enabling chiropractors to tailor treatments to the specific needs and goals of each patient.

Marketing and Patient Acquisition

Beyond practice management and patient care, some chiropractic software solutions offer marketing tools designed to help practices grow their patient base. These may include features for managing social media, email marketing campaigns, and patient reviews, helping to attract new patients and retain existing ones.

Conclusion

Utilizing chiropractic software is essential for modern chiropractic practices aiming to enhance efficiency, improve patient care, and navigate the complexities of healthcare management. By leveraging the power of technology, chiropractors can optimize their practice operations, engage more effectively with patients, and focus on delivering high-quality chiropractic care.

9.3 Telehealth and Digital Patient Engagement

The integration of telehealth and digital patient engagement tools into chiropractic practice marks a significant shift towards a more accessible, patient-centered model of care. These technologies enable continuous communication and care delivery, breaking down geographical barriers and offering convenience to both patients and healthcare providers.

Telehealth in Chiropractic Care

Telehealth, or telemedicine, involves the use of digital communication tools to conduct healthcare consultations and services remotely. In chiropractic care, telehealth can be particularly useful for initial consultations, follow-up appointments, patient education, and management of chronic conditions. While the hands-on nature of chiropractic adjustments requires in-person visits, many aspects of patient care and support can be effectively delivered through telehealth platforms.

- **Benefits:** Telehealth provides patients with easier access to care, particularly those in remote areas or with mobility challenges. It also offers flexibility in scheduling and reduces the time and costs associated with travel. For chiropractors, telehealth can expand the patient base and improve efficiency in care delivery.

Digital Patient Engagement Tools

Digital patient engagement tools are designed to foster an ongoing, interactive relationship between patients and healthcare providers. These tools include patient portals, mobile health apps, wearable technology, and automated communication systems for reminders and health tips.

- **Patient Portals:** Secure online platforms that give patients 24/7 access to their personal health information, appointment scheduling, prescription renewals, and direct communication with their healthcare provider.

- **Mobile Health Apps:** Apps that provide health information, track progress towards health goals, and offer reminders for medication and appointments.

- **Wearable Technology:** Devices that monitor health metrics such as physical activity, sleep patterns, and heart rate, allowing patients and chiropractors to track improvements or identify areas needing attention.

- **Automated Communication Systems:** Systems that send out reminders for appointments, follow-ups, and health maintenance tips, keeping patients engaged in their healthcare journey.

Implementing Telehealth and Engagement Tools

Implementing these technologies requires consideration of several factors:

- **Privacy and Security:** Ensuring compliance with health information privacy regulations and securing patient data is paramount.

- **Technology Training:** Both staff and patients may require training to effectively use telehealth and engagement platforms.

- **Integration with Existing Systems:** Telehealth and engagement tools should be integrated with the clinic's existing EHR and practice management systems for seamless operation.

- **Patient Accessibility:** Consideration should be given to the digital literacy and access to technology among the clinic's patient population to ensure that telehealth options are inclusive.

Conclusion

Telehealth and digital patient engagement represent the future of chiropractic care, offering a blend of convenience, efficiency, and enhanced patient experience. By adopting these technologies, chiropractic practices can not only meet the evolving expectations of their patients but also improve health outcomes through better communication, monitoring, and patient involvement in their own care.

9.4 Exercise: 10 MCQs with Answers at the End

1. What is the primary benefit of integrating Electronic Health Records (EHR) into chiropractic practice?

   A) Reducing physical activity

   B) Centralizing patient information

   C) Increasing paper usage

   D) Decreasing patient interaction

2. Chiropractic software often includes what feature for enhancing practice management?

   A) Manual appointment booking only

   B) Automated billing and coding suggestions

   C) Paper-based patient records

   D) Decreased data security

3. What does patient engagement tools in chiropractic software aim to improve?

   A) Patient confusion

   B) Communication and satisfaction

   C) Patient wait times

   D) Costs for patients

4. Why is telehealth becoming an important part of chiropractic care?

A) It reduces the quality of care

B) It limits patient access to services

C) It extends the reach of chiropractic care

D) It increases the need for in-person visits

5. What advantage does digital patient engagement offer?

A) Decreases patient involvement in their care

B) Enhances patient communication and empowerment

C) Complicates appointment scheduling

D) Reduces practice efficiency

6. How does utilizing chiropractic software benefit billing and insurance processing?

A) By making the process more error-prone

B) Through streamlined and automated processes

C) Increasing manual paperwork

D) Slowing down reimbursement

7. Which is a feature of modern chiropractic software for clinical documentation?

A) Fixed templates only

B) Customizable forms and templates

C) Handwritten notes only

D) No option for digital storage

8. Telehealth capabilities in chiropractic software allow for:

A) Only local patient consultations

B) Decreased patient engagement

C) Virtual consultations

D) Reducing the quality of patient care

9. Marketing tools in chiropractic software help practices to:

A) Reduce patient base

B) Attract and retain patients

C) Ignore digital marketing strategies

D) Increase advertising costs

10. What is the goal of customizable treatment plans in chiropractic software?

A) To provide a generic approach to care

B) To tailor treatments to individual patient needs

C) To complicate treatment planning

D) To limit chiropractor intervention

Answers:

1. B) Centralizing patient information

2. B) Automated billing and coding suggestions

3. B) Communication and satisfaction

4. C) It extends the reach of chiropractic care

5. B) Enhances patient communication and empowerment

6. B) Through streamlined and automated processes

7. B) Customizable forms and templates

8. C) Virtual consultations

9. B) Attract and retain patients

10. B) To tailor treatments to individual patient needs

Chapter 10: Managing Chiropractic Supplies and Equipment

10.1 Inventory Management Best Practices

Effective inventory management is crucial for the smooth operation of chiropractic practices. It ensures that essential supplies and equipment are always available to provide the best care to patients without interruption. Implementing best practices in inventory management can lead to cost savings, improved efficiency, and enhanced patient satisfaction.

Regular Inventory Audits

Conduct regular audits to track the quantities of supplies and condition of equipment. This helps in identifying any discrepancies between recorded and actual inventory levels, allowing for timely adjustments.

Implement an Inventory Management System

Utilizing a digital inventory management system can streamline the tracking and ordering process. These systems can automate reorder alerts when stock levels reach a predetermined threshold, ensuring that supplies are replenished before running out.

Categorize Supplies and Equipment

Organize inventory into categories based on type, usage frequency, and expiration dates. This categorization simplifies the process of locating and tracking items, making inventory management more efficient.

Establish Reorder Points

Set minimum stock levels for each item to determine when to reorder. These reorder points should consider lead times for ordering and receiving supplies, as well as fluctuations in patient volume that may affect usage rates.

Negotiate with Suppliers

Build relationships with suppliers to negotiate better prices, bulk purchase discounts, or more favorable terms. A good relationship with suppliers can also lead to better service and reliability.

Optimize Storage Solutions

Effective storage solutions maximize space, preserve the condition of supplies and equipment, and keep items organized and accessible. Consider the specific storage requirements for different items, such as temperature controls for sensitive materials.

Monitor Usage Trends

Tracking the usage trends of supplies and equipment can provide insights into patient demand and help in forecasting future needs. This information can inform purchasing decisions and prevent overstocking or stockouts.

Train Staff on Inventory Management Practices

Ensure all staff members are trained on inventory management procedures, including proper storage, tracking, and ordering practices. Staff training promotes accountability and consistency in managing inventory.

Review and Adjust Inventory Practices Regularly

Inventory needs and challenges can evolve, requiring regular review and adjustment of inventory practices. Stay adaptable and seek continuous improvement to optimize inventory management strategies over time.

Conclusion

Adopting best practices in inventory management is essential for maintaining the operational efficiency of chiropractic practices. By ensuring that the right supplies and equipment are available when needed, practices can provide uninterrupted, high-quality care to their patients. Effective inventory management also contributes to cost control and the overall success of the practice.

10.2 Maintenance of Chiropractic Equipment

Maintaining chiropractic equipment is essential for ensuring the safety and effectiveness of treatments offered to patients. Proper maintenance routines not only extend the lifespan of equipment but also safeguard against potential malfunctions that could impact patient care. Here are key practices for maintaining chiropractic equipment effectively.

Regular Inspection and Calibration

Conduct regular inspections of all chiropractic equipment to check for wear and tear, operational issues, or any signs of damage. Certain pieces of equipment, like adjustment tables and electronic instruments, may require calibration to ensure they are providing accurate readings and functioning correctly. Setting a schedule for these inspections and calibrations helps prevent issues from going unnoticed.

Cleanliness and Disinfection

Maintaining cleanliness is crucial for patient safety and the longevity of equipment. Regular cleaning and disinfection of surfaces, especially those that come into direct contact with patients, prevent the spread of infection and maintain a hygienic practice environment. Use appropriate cleaning agents that are effective yet safe for the equipment materials.

Follow Manufacturer's Guidelines

Always refer to the manufacturer's maintenance guidelines for specific care instructions for each piece of equipment. These guidelines provide valuable information on cleaning procedures, recommended maintenance schedules, and troubleshooting tips. Adhering to these recommendations ensures the equipment is maintained correctly and operates as intended.

Prompt Repairs and Servicing

Address any signs of malfunction or damage immediately. Delaying repairs can lead to further damage or equipment failure, potentially causing interruptions in patient care or even safety risks. Use qualified technicians for servicing and repairs to ensure the work is done correctly and to maintain any warranties.

Record Keeping

Keep detailed records of all maintenance activities, including inspections, calibrations, cleaning, and repairs. These records help track the maintenance history of each piece of equipment, identify recurring issues, and make informed decisions about replacements or upgrades.

Staff Training

Ensure that all staff members who use or are responsible for the equipment are trained in proper operation, basic troubleshooting, and maintenance procedures. Knowledgeable staff can help prevent equipment misuse, which is a common cause of wear and tear.

Invest in Quality Equipment Covers and Protectors

Using covers and protectors can shield equipment from spills, dust, and other environmental factors that could cause damage over time. These protective accessories are particularly important for delicate instruments and electronic devices.

Budget for Maintenance and Upgrades

Allocate funds in the practice's budget for regular maintenance and potential equipment upgrades. Investing in maintenance and staying updated with the latest equipment technology can enhance treatment efficiency and patient satisfaction.

Conclusion

Effective maintenance of chiropractic equipment is a critical aspect of practice management. It ensures that treatments are performed safely and effectively, contributing to the overall success of the practice. By implementing regular maintenance routines, adhering to manufacturer guidelines, and investing in staff training, chiropractic practices can maintain their equipment in optimal condition, providing the highest standard of care to their patients.

10.3 Ordering and Stocking Supplies Efficiently

Efficient ordering and stocking of supplies are critical components of successful chiropractic practice management.

Properly managed inventory ensures that the necessary supplies are always on hand to provide uninterrupted patient care, while also controlling costs and minimizing waste. Here are strategies to enhance efficiency in ordering and stocking chiropractic supplies.

Understand Your Practice's Needs

Begin by assessing the specific needs of your practice. Consider the types of treatments offered, patient volume, and any seasonal variations in demand. This understanding will help you determine which supplies are needed regularly and in what quantities.

Utilize an Automated Inventory Management System

An automated inventory management system can significantly streamline the ordering and stocking process. These systems track inventory levels in real-time, automatically generate reorder alerts when supplies reach critical levels, and can even automate the ordering process with pre-approved suppliers, reducing the risk of stockouts or overordering.

Establish Strong Relationships with Suppliers

Developing strong relationships with reliable suppliers is key to efficient inventory management. Trusted suppliers can offer valuable insights into product availability, lead times, and potential alternatives for backordered items. They may also provide priority service, volume discounts, or flexible return policies, further enhancing efficiency and cost-effectiveness.

Implement Just-in-Time (JIT) Inventory Practices

Just-in-Time (JIT) inventory practices involve ordering supplies as close as possible to when they are actually needed. This approach can reduce inventory costs and minimize the storage space required. However, it requires accurate demand forecasting and reliable suppliers to avoid potential disruptions in patient care.

Regularly Review and Adjust Order Quantities

Regularly review your ordering patterns and adjust quantities based on actual usage and changing needs. This ongoing adjustment process helps prevent both overstocking, which ties up capital and storage space, and understocking, which can disrupt patient care.

Standardize Products Where Possible

Standardizing supplies and equipment across your practice can simplify ordering, reduce costs, and minimize training requirements for staff. Using fewer, well-chosen products can also simplify inventory management and improve bargaining power with suppliers.

Train Staff on Inventory Best Practices

Ensure that all staff members are trained on inventory best practices, including how to properly use inventory management systems, store supplies, and monitor expiration dates. A well-informed team can contribute significantly to the efficiency and accuracy of inventory management.

Monitor and Adjust for Seasonal Variations

Be aware of and plan for seasonal variations in patient volume and supply needs. Adjust ordering patterns to accommodate anticipated changes, ensuring that your practice is well-prepared for busier periods without overstocking during slower times.

Conclusion

Efficient ordering and stocking of supplies are fundamental to the smooth operation of a chiropractic practice. By leveraging technology, maintaining strong supplier relationships, and implementing smart inventory strategies, practices can ensure they have the necessary supplies on hand to meet patient needs while also controlling costs and optimizing storage space.

10.4 Exercise: 10 MCQs with Answers at the End

1. What is the primary goal of effective inventory management in chiropractic practices?

   A) To minimize patient care

   B) To ensure necessary supplies are always available

   C) To increase storage needs

   D) To complicate ordering processes

2. An automated inventory management system helps by:

A) Increasing manual record-keeping

B) Automatically generating reorder alerts

C) Reducing inventory visibility

D) Limiting access to inventory data

3. Building strong relationships with suppliers can lead to:

A) Higher supply costs

B) Reduced service reliability

C) Volume discounts and flexible return policies

D) Longer lead times for orders

4. Just-in-Time (JIT) inventory practices aim to:

A) Increase inventory costs

B) Order supplies well in advance

C) Order supplies as close as possible to when they are needed

D) Stockpile supplies

5. Regularly reviewing and adjusting order quantities is important because it:

A) Prevents any adjustments to inventory levels

B) Increases the risk of stockouts

C) Helps prevent overstocking and understocking

D) Guarantees permanent inventory surplus

6. Standardizing products across a practice can:

A) Complicate inventory management

B) Increase the need for diverse storage solutions

C) Reduce costs and simplify ordering

D) Decrease bargaining power with suppliers

7. Training staff on inventory best practices is crucial for:

A) Decreasing inventory accuracy

B) Limiting staff involvement in inventory management

C) Enhancing efficiency and accuracy of inventory management

D) Encouraging independent inventory management practices

8. Seasonal variations in patient volume:

A) Should not influence ordering patterns

B) Require adjustments to ordering patterns to prevent overstocking or understocking

C) Are irrelevant to chiropractic practices

D) Decrease the need for inventory management

9. The primary benefit of utilizing an automated inventory management system is to:

A) Avoid using technology in the practice

B) Manually track all inventory items

C) Streamline the tracking and ordering process

D) Increase the time spent on inventory management

10. Effective inventory management in chiropractic practices leads to:

A) Disruptions in patient care

B) Increased operational costs

C) Improved patient satisfaction and cost control

D) A reduction in the variety of supplies used

Answers:

1. B) To ensure necessary supplies are always available

2. B) Automatically generating reorder alerts

3. C) Volume discounts and flexible return policies

4. C) Order supplies as close as possible to when they are needed

5. C) Helps prevent overstocking and understocking

6. C) Reduce costs and simplify ordering

7. C) Enhancing efficiency and accuracy of inventory management

8. B) Require adjustments to ordering patterns to prevent overstocking or understocking

9. C) Streamline the tracking and ordering process

10. C) Improved patient satisfaction and cost control

Chapter 11: Safety Protocols in the Chiropractic Office

11.1 Understanding and Implementing Occupational Safety and Health Administration Guidelines

Ensuring a safe and healthy work environment is a paramount concern for chiropractic offices. Adhering to guidelines set by the leading national public health institute focused on occupational safety significantly contributes to protecting both staff and patients from potential health hazards.

Comprehending Workplace Safety Standards

These standards encompass a wide range of protocols designed to minimize risks associated with physical injuries, biological hazards, and environmental factors within healthcare settings. Understanding these guidelines is the first step in creating a safer chiropractic practice.

Risk Assessment and Management

Performing regular risk assessments to identify potential hazards in the office is essential. This process involves examining all aspects of the practice, from patient treatment areas to employee workstations, to identify where improvements can be made to enhance safety.

Implementing Control Measures

Once risks have been identified, appropriate control measures should be put in place. This may include ergonomic adjustments to furniture and equipment, proper handling and disposal of sharp objects, and the use of personal protective equipment (PPE) when necessary.

Maintaining Cleanliness and Hygiene

Maintaining a high standard of cleanliness and hygiene is crucial in preventing the spread of infection. Regular cleaning and disinfection of treatment areas, equipment, and communal spaces are required, with particular attention to high-touch surfaces.

Staff Training and Education

Ensuring that all staff members are adequately trained in occupational safety and health practices is vital. This includes education on the correct use of PPE, emergency procedures, and the importance of maintaining a clean and safe work environment.

Emergency Preparedness

Having a well-defined plan for emergencies, including potential injuries, fires, or biological exposures, is crucial. This plan should be readily accessible to all staff members and include clear instructions on what to do in various emergency situations.

Record Keeping and Documentation

Maintaining accurate records of safety inspections, incident reports, and training activities is required for compliance and continuous improvement. These records can also provide valuable insights into areas where safety protocols may need to be enhanced.

Engaging Staff and Patients in Safety Protocols

Creating a culture of safety within the chiropractic office involves engaging both staff and patients. Encouraging feedback and suggestions for improving safety measures can lead to more effective and comprehensive safety protocols.

Regular Review and Update of Safety Procedures

Safety protocols should be regularly reviewed and updated to reflect changes in regulations, new health and safety research, and the evolving needs of the practice. Continuous improvement in safety practices ensures the well-being of both staff and patients.

Conclusion

Implementing guidelines from the leading national public health institute focused on occupational safety is fundamental to the operation of a safe and efficient chiropractic office. By understanding and applying these guidelines, chiropractic practices can mitigate risks, ensure compliance with regulations, and provide a secure environment for both patients and employees.

11.2 Infection Control and Hygiene Practices

In chiropractic offices, as in all healthcare settings, infection control and hygiene practices are critical components of patient care and staff safety. Effective measures can significantly reduce the risk of infection transmission, ensuring a safe environment for both patients and healthcare providers.

Hand Hygiene

Regular and thorough hand washing is the cornerstone of preventing infection spread. Staff should wash their hands with soap and water or use an alcohol-based hand sanitizer before and after each patient contact, after handling waste, and when hands are visibly soiled.

Personal Protective Equipment (PPE)

The appropriate use of PPE, such as gloves, masks, and eye protection, provides a barrier against infections. Staff should be trained on the correct use, removal, and disposal of PPE, especially when dealing with bodily fluids or when in close contact with patients showing signs of infectious diseases.

Surface Disinfection

Regular cleaning and disinfection of surfaces and equipment in treatment areas are essential. High-touch surfaces, including treatment tables, door handles, and reception counters, require frequent disinfection with EPA-registered disinfectants effective against a broad range of pathogens.

Sterilization of Reusable Equipment

Any reusable equipment that comes into contact with patients should be properly cleaned and sterilized according to established protocols. This includes instruments used in manual therapy or any other treatment modalities that require direct patient contact.

Management of Waste

Proper waste management protocols should be followed, especially for the disposal of sharps and other potentially infectious materials. Sharps containers should be used to prevent needle-stick injuries, and biohazard waste should be disposed of in accordance with local regulations.

Air Quality and Ventilation

Maintaining good air quality and proper ventilation reduces the risk of airborne infections. The use of HEPA filters, regular maintenance of HVAC systems, and ensuring natural ventilation where possible can help achieve this.

Patient Screening and Scheduling

Screening patients for symptoms of infectious diseases before appointments can help prevent the spread of infections within the office. Consider rescheduling patients who exhibit symptoms or have been exposed to infectious diseases, and implement telehealth services where appropriate.

Education and Training

Ongoing education and training for all staff on infection control practices and updates on guidelines from health authorities are crucial. This includes understanding the modes of transmission, the importance of vaccination, and strategies for managing outbreaks.

Patient Education

Educating patients on the importance of hygiene practices, including hand hygiene and respiratory etiquette, can further reduce the risk of infection transmission. Providing hand sanitizer stations and educational materials in the waiting area can promote these practices.

Conclusion

Implementing robust infection control and hygiene practices in chiropractic offices is essential for safeguarding health and preventing the spread of infections. By adhering to these guidelines, chiropractic practices can maintain a safe and healthy environment for patients and staff alike.

11.3 Emergency Preparedness and Response

Preparedness for emergencies within a chiropractic office is essential to safeguarding the health and safety of both patients and staff. An effective emergency response plan can mitigate risks and ensure a coordinated response to various situations, from medical emergencies to natural disasters.

Developing an Emergency Response Plan

Creating a comprehensive emergency response plan is the first step. This plan should address a wide range of potential emergencies, including medical incidents, fire, natural disasters, and security threats. It should outline specific actions to take in each scenario, including evacuation routes, emergency contact numbers, and procedures for administering first aid.

Staff Training and Drills

Regular training sessions for all staff members on the emergency response plan are crucial. This training should cover basic first aid, CPR, the use of emergency equipment, and evacuation procedures. Conducting regular drills can help staff become familiar with emergency protocols, reducing panic and confusion during actual emergencies.

Emergency Equipment and Supplies

Ensuring that emergency equipment and supplies are readily available and well-maintained is vital. This includes first aid kits, automated external defibrillators (AEDs), fire extinguishers, and emergency lighting. Regular checks should be performed to ensure that all equipment is in working order and that supplies are not expired.

Communication Systems

Effective communication systems are essential for alerting staff and patients to emergencies and coordinating a response. This may involve alarm systems, public address systems, and having a list of emergency contact numbers readily available, including local emergency services, poison control, and utility companies.

Patient Safety Measures

During emergencies, patient safety is a top priority. The emergency response plan should include procedures for safely evacitating patients, especially those with mobility issues or other vulnerabilities. Staff should be trained on how to assist patients in an emergency and ensure that everyone is accounted for.

Coordination with Local Emergency Services

Establishing a relationship with local emergency services can enhance the effectiveness of the emergency response. Informing local fire, police, and medical services about the clinic's location, layout, and specific risks can facilitate a more efficient and coordinated response when emergencies occur.

Documentation and Debriefing

Following any emergency, documenting the event, actions taken, and any injuries or damages is important for insurance purposes, regulatory compliance, and learning. A debriefing session with staff to review the response and identify areas for improvement can enhance future preparedness.

Regular Review and Update of the Emergency Plan

The emergency response plan should be regularly reviewed and updated to reflect changes in the practice, staff, or local emergency services. New threats or lessons learned from drills or actual events may also necessitate updates to the plan.

Conclusion

Emergency preparedness and response in a chiropractic office are critical components of practice management. By developing a comprehensive emergency plan, training staff, maintaining necessary equipment, and establishing communication with local emergency services, chiropractic practices can ensure a safe environment for patients and staff alike.

11.4 Exercise: 10 MCQs with Answers at the End

1. What is the primary purpose of an emergency response plan in a chiropractic office?

A) To complicate daily operations

B) To safeguard health and safety during emergencies

C) To increase paperwork

D) To limit staff responsibilities

2. Regular staff training on emergency protocols is crucial for:

A) Reducing the effectiveness of response

B) Increasing panic during emergencies

C) Ensuring familiarity with emergency procedures

D) Decreasing staff confidence

3. Which equipment should be readily available and well-maintained for emergencies?

A) Decorative items

B) First aid kits and automated external defibrillators (AEDs)

C) Non-essential office supplies

D) Outdated technology

4. Effective communication systems during emergencies are essential for:

A) Creating confusion

B) Alerting and coordinating staff and patient response

C) Ignoring emergencies

D) Delaying response time

5. The emergency response plan should include procedures for:

A) Safely evacuating only the staff

B) Keeping patients uninformed

C) Safely evacuating patients, especially those with vulnerabilities

D) Ignoring local emergency services

6. Establishing a relationship with local emergency services can:

A) Complicate responses

B) Reduce the effectiveness of local services

C) Enhance the coordination and efficiency of the emergency response

D) Discourage clinic staff from responding to emergencies

7. Following an emergency, it's important to:

A) Ignore the event

B) Document the event and review the response

C) Avoid discussing the event with staff

D) Immediately forget the incident

8. Regular review and update of the emergency plan are needed to:

A) Maintain outdated procedures

B) Reflect changes in the practice and staff

C) Decrease the plan's relevance

D) Ignore new threats

9. Conducting regular drills helps:

A) Increase the likelihood of errors during an actual emergency

B) Familiarize staff with emergency protocols

C) Discourage participation in emergency preparedness

D) Reduce the need for an emergency plan

10. An emergency response plan should address:

A) Only minor incidents

B) A wide range of potential emergencies

C) Events that are highly unlikely to occur

D) Only the specific interests of the clinic owner

Answers:

1. B) To safeguard health and safety during emergencies

2. C) Ensuring familiarity with emergency procedures

3. B) First aid kits and automated external defibrillators (AEDs)

4. B) Alerting and coordinating staff and patient response

5. C) Safely evacuating patients, especially those with vulnerabilities

6. C) Enhance the coordination and efficiency of the emergency response

7. B) Document the event and review the response

8. B) Reflect changes in the practice and staff

9. B) Familiarize staff with emergency protocols

10. B) A wide range of potential emergencies

Chapter 12: Financial Management for Chiropractic Assistants

12.1 Billing and Insurance Processing

For chiropractic assistants, mastering the intricacies of billing and insurance processing is crucial for the financial health of the practice. Efficient and accurate billing practices ensure timely reimbursements from insurance companies and patients, contributing to the clinic's overall financial stability.

Understanding Insurance Policies and Coverage

A deep understanding of various insurance policies, including private health insurance and government-sponsored programs, is essential. Chiropractic assistants should familiarize themselves with the coverage details, limitations, and exclusions of different plans to accurately process claims and inform patients of their financial responsibilities.

Accurate Coding and Documentation

The accuracy of coding and documentation cannot be overstated in billing and insurance processing. Using the correct codes for diagnoses and treatments (such as CPT, ICD-10, and

HCPCS codes) is critical for claims acceptance. Regular training and updates on coding standards are vital for staying compliant and minimizing claim denials or delays.

Efficient Claim Submission and Follow-up

Timely submission of insurance claims and diligent follow-up are key to ensuring prompt payments. Establishing a systematic process for tracking claim statuses, identifying and rectifying denied or rejected claims, and appealing decisions when necessary helps maintain a steady cash flow.

Patient Billing and Communication

Clear and transparent communication with patients about their billing and insurance benefits is important. Providing detailed invoices, explaining out-of-pocket costs, and offering flexible payment options can enhance patient satisfaction and reduce the incidence of unpaid bills.

Utilizing Billing Software

Investing in specialized billing software can streamline the billing and insurance processing workflow. These systems can automate many aspects of the process, from claim generation and submission to tracking and reporting, improving efficiency and accuracy.

Staying Updated with Insurance Regulations

Insurance regulations and healthcare laws are continually evolving. Keeping abreast of changes that affect billing practices and insurance claim processing is necessary to ensure compliance and optimize reimbursement rates.

Handling Patient Inquiries and Disputes

Chiropractic assistants often serve as the first point of contact for patients with billing inquiries or disputes. Handling these interactions with patience, empathy, and professionalism can resolve concerns effectively and maintain positive patient relations.

Regular Audits and Compliance Checks

Conducting regular audits of billing practices and compliance with insurance regulations helps identify areas for improvement and prevent potential legal and financial issues. These audits can be internal or performed by external consultants specializing in healthcare billing compliance.

Conclusion

Billing and insurance processing are critical components of financial management in chiropractic practices. By developing a comprehensive understanding of insurance policies, maintaining accuracy in coding and documentation, and employing efficient billing practices, chiropractic assistants can significantly contribute to the financial success and sustainability of the practice.

12.2 Financial Policies and Patient Billing

Effective financial management is essential in chiropractic practices, not only for sustaining the business but also for maintaining transparency and trust with patients. Establishing clear financial policies and handling patient billing with care are key components of this process.

Developing Clear Financial Policies

Creating comprehensive financial policies provides a framework for all monetary transactions within the practice. These policies should cover payment expectations, insurance billing, options for uninsured or underinsured patients, and procedures for handling overdue accounts. Clearly stated policies help avoid misunderstandings and ensure that both staff and patients are aware of their financial responsibilities.

Communication of Financial Responsibilities

Communicating financial responsibilities to patients before the commencement of treatment is crucial. Patients should be informed about their coverage, any out-of-pocket costs, and the payment options available to them. Transparent communication upfront can prevent billing surprises and foster a trusting relationship between the practice and its patients.

Insurance Verification and Billing

Verifying a patient's insurance coverage before providing services can significantly streamline the billing process. Understanding the extent of coverage, co-pays, deductibles, and any services not covered by insurance allows the practice to bill accurately and reduces the likelihood of disputes. Efficient insurance processing, including timely submission of claims and thorough follow-up, is vital for maintaining cash flow.

Flexible Payment Options

Offering flexible payment options, such as payment plans for high-cost treatments, can make chiropractic care more accessible to a broader range of patients. It's important to manage these arrangements carefully to ensure they are fair and that they do not adversely affect the practice's financial health.

Handling Billing Disputes and Inquiries

Prompt and courteous handling of billing disputes and inquiries reinforces the practice's commitment to patient satisfaction and can prevent minor issues from escalating. Staff should be trained to address these concerns professionally, offering clear explanations and, where necessary, adjustments to billing.

Use of Billing Software

Utilizing specialized billing software can automate many aspects of the financial management process, from generating invoices to tracking payments and managing accounts receivable. This technology can reduce errors, save time, and provide valuable insights into the practice's financial performance.

Regular Financial Reviews

Regular reviews of the practice's financial policies and billing procedures ensure that they remain effective and compliant with any changes in healthcare laws and insurance regulations. These reviews can also identify opportunities for improving financial management and patient satisfaction.

Conclusion

Financial policies and patient billing are critical aspects of financial management in chiropractic practices. By establishing clear policies, communicating effectively with patients, efficiently managing insurance processing, and leveraging technology, practices can ensure financial stability while maintaining positive relationships with their patients.

12.3 Budgeting and Financial Planning for the Clinic

Effective financial management is crucial for the sustainability and growth of any chiropractic clinic. Budgeting and financial planning are key components of this process, enabling the clinic to allocate resources efficiently, plan for future growth, and ensure financial stability.

Understanding Clinic Expenses

The first step in budgeting is to comprehensively understand the clinic's expenses. These can be divided into fixed costs (such as rent, utilities, and salaries) and variable costs (including supplies, equipment maintenance, and marketing expenses). Accurate tracking of these expenses is essential for effective budgeting.

Revenue Forecasting

Accurately forecasting revenue is challenging but essential. Consider factors such as the number of patients, average revenue per patient, and seasonal fluctuations in business. Historical data can provide a basis for these forecasts, but it's also important to consider potential changes in the market or service offerings.

Setting Financial Goals

Financial goals should be specific, measurable, achievable, relevant, and time-bound (SMART). Goals might include increasing patient numbers, expanding services, or saving for new equipment. These goals should guide the budgeting process and inform financial decisions.

Allocating Resources Wisely

Resource allocation involves deciding how to distribute available funds across various areas of the clinic. Prioritize spending on areas that directly contribute to patient care and revenue generation, such as marketing to attract new patients or investing in staff training and development.

Emergency Fund

Setting aside funds for unexpected expenses or downturns in business is a prudent financial strategy. An emergency fund can help the clinic navigate through tough times without compromising patient care or employee salaries.

Investment in Growth

Part of financial planning involves investing in the clinic's growth. This could include expanding the physical space, investing in new technology, or adding new services. These investments should be carefully planned and aligned with the clinic's long-term strategic goals.

Regular Financial Review

Regularly reviewing the clinic's financial performance against the budget can help identify areas where adjustments may be needed. This could involve cutting unnecessary expenses, adjusting pricing strategies, or identifying new revenue opportunities.

Professional Financial Advice

Seeking professional financial advice can be beneficial, especially when dealing with complex financial planning, tax obligations, or significant investments. A financial advisor with experience in healthcare can provide valuable insights and guidance.

Conclusion

Budgeting and financial planning are essential for the effective management of a chiropractic clinic. By understanding expenses, forecasting revenue, setting financial goals, and allocating resources wisely, clinics can ensure financial health and support their long-term vision and growth. Regular financial review and professional advice can further enhance financial stability and success.

12.4 Exercise: 10 MCQs with Answers at the End

1. What is the primary purpose of budgeting and financial planning in a chiropractic clinic?

   A) To limit the growth of the clinic

   B) To ensure financial stability and plan for future growth

   C) To complicate financial management

   D) To reduce staff salaries

2. Which type of cost remains constant regardless of the number of patients seen in the clinic?

   A) Variable costs

   B) Fixed costs

   C) Incidental costs

D) Deferred costs

3. What is important to consider when forecasting revenue for a chiropractic clinic?

A) Only the previous month's revenue

B) The number of patients and average revenue per patient

C) Ignoring seasonal fluctuations

D) Setting unrealistic revenue targets

4. Setting financial goals for a clinic should follow which criteria?

A) Vague and unmeasurable

B) Specific, Measurable, Achievable, Relevant, Time-bound (SMART)

C) Unachievable and irrelevant

D) Not time-bound

5. How should resources be allocated in a chiropractic clinic?

A) Randomly, without prioritization

B) Based on the clinic owner's personal preferences

C) Prioritizing areas that contribute to patient care and revenue generation

D) Solely on new office decor

6. Why is having an emergency fund important for a chiropractic clinic?

A) It is not necessary for healthcare facilities

B) To cover unexpected expenses or downturns in business

C) Only for aesthetic updates to the clinic

D) To decrease overall financial stability

7. Investments in the growth of a chiropractic clinic could include:

A) Reducing the number of services offered

B) Expanding the physical space or adding new services

C) Ignoring new technology

D) Decreasing marketing efforts

8. Regular financial review helps to:

A) Ignore financial issues

B) Identify areas where adjustments may be needed

C) Increase unnecessary expenses

D) Set unrealistic financial goals

9. Seeking professional financial advice is beneficial for:

A) Only small clinics

B) Making simple financial decisions

C) Dealing with complex financial planning and investments

D) Reducing the credibility of the clinic

10. Fixed costs in a chiropractic clinic typically include:

   A) Supplies used per patient

   B) Rent, utilities, and salaries

   C) Marketing expenses

   D) Cost of goods sold

Answers:

1. B) To ensure financial stability and plan for future growth

2. B) Fixed costs

3. B) The number of patients and average revenue per patient

4. B) Specific, Measurable, Achievable, Relevant, Time-bound (SMART)

5. C) Prioritizing areas that contribute to patient care and revenue generation

6. B) To cover unexpected expenses or downturns in business

7. B) Expanding the physical space or adding new services

8. B) Identify areas where adjustments may be needed

9. C) Dealing with complex financial planning and investments

10. B) Rent, utilities, and salaries

Chapter 13: Leadership and Teamwork in the Chiropractic Setting

13.1 Cultivating Leadership Skills

Effective leadership is crucial in any chiropractic setting, influencing the clinic's culture, operational efficiency, and the quality of patient care. Cultivating leadership skills within this context involves developing qualities and practices that inspire, guide, and support the team towards achieving shared goals.

Self-awareness and Emotional Intelligence

Understanding one's strengths, weaknesses, and emotional triggers is the foundation of strong leadership. Leaders with high emotional intelligence can manage their emotions and understand those of others, facilitating better communication and conflict resolution within the team.

Vision and Strategic Thinking

Effective leaders possess a clear vision for the clinic's future and the strategic thinking necessary to guide their team towards these goals. This involves setting clear objectives, planning for long-term success, and adapting to changes in the healthcare landscape.

Communication Skills

Leaders must be able to communicate effectively with their team, conveying ideas clearly and listening to feedback. Open and honest communication fosters trust, encourages collaboration, and ensures that everyone is aligned with the clinic's objectives.

Empowering and Developing Others

A key aspect of leadership is the ability to empower and develop team members. This includes providing opportunities for professional growth, delegating responsibilities that stretch their capabilities, and offering constructive feedback to help them improve.

Team Building and Collaboration

Cultivating a strong team dynamic is essential for a productive work environment. Leaders should encourage collaboration, recognize individual and team achievements, and address any issues that may affect team cohesion.

Decision Making and Problem Solving

Leaders are often required to make difficult decisions and solve complex problems. Developing these skills involves gathering information, considering various perspectives, weighing the potential outcomes, and making choices that are in the best interest of the clinic and its patients.

Adaptability and Resilience

The ability to adapt to changing circumstances and overcome challenges is a hallmark of effective leadership. Leaders must remain flexible, learn from setbacks, and maintain a positive attitude even in difficult situations.

Ethical Conduct and Integrity

Leaders in the chiropractic setting must uphold the highest standards of ethical conduct and integrity. This includes being honest, treating others with respect, and making decisions that reflect the clinic's values and commitment to patient care.

Mentorship and Role Modeling

Serving as a mentor and role model for the team is an important part of leadership. By exemplifying the qualities and behaviors expected of others, leaders can inspire their team to strive for excellence in their work and professional conduct.

Conclusion

Cultivating leadership skills within a chiropractic setting enhances the clinic's operational effectiveness, team morale, and patient care quality. By focusing on personal development, strategic thinking, and team dynamics, chiropractic professionals can lead their practices towards success and fulfillment.

13.2 Effective Team Communication

Effective communication within a chiropractic team is essential for delivering high-quality patient care, maintaining a positive work environment, and achieving the clinic's operational goals. It encompasses not just the exchange of information, but also the ability to listen, understand, and respond in ways that promote teamwork and mutual respect.

Open and Transparent Communication

Creating a culture of open and transparent communication encourages team members to share ideas, concerns, and feedback freely. This environment fosters trust and helps prevent misunderstandings that could lead to conflicts or errors in patient care.

Regular Team Meetings

Holding regular team meetings provides a structured opportunity for staff to discuss clinic operations, patient care issues, and any other relevant topics. These meetings should be inclusive, allowing every team member to voice their opinions and contribute to decision-making processes.

Active Listening

Active listening involves paying full attention to the speaker, understanding their message, and responding thoughtfully. By practicing active listening, team members can improve mutual understanding and collaboration, ensuring that everyone feels heard and valued.

Non-Verbal Communication

Non-verbal cues, such as body language and facial expressions, play a significant role in communication. Being aware of and responsive to these cues can enhance understanding and empathy within the team, contributing to a more cohesive work environment.

Clear and Concise Messaging

Communicating in a clear and concise manner helps prevent confusion and ensures that important information is understood by all team members. This is particularly crucial when discussing patient care plans, treatment protocols, or emergency procedures.

Feedback and Constructive Criticism

Providing constructive feedback is vital for personal and professional growth. Feedback should be specific, objective, and delivered in a manner that encourages improvement rather than defensiveness. Likewise, receiving feedback with an open mind is important for continuous learning and development.

Conflict Resolution Skills

Conflicts can arise in any team, but effective communication is key to resolving them constructively. Approaching conflicts with a focus on finding mutually beneficial solutions, rather than assigning blame, can help maintain positive team dynamics.

Utilizing Technology for Communication

Technology, such as email, messaging apps, and project management tools, can enhance team communication, especially for coordinating tasks and sharing information. However, it's important to balance digital communication with face-to-face interactions to preserve personal connections within the team.

Cultural Competence

In diverse teams, being culturally competent — understanding and respecting differences in backgrounds, beliefs, and communication styles — is crucial for effective communication. This awareness can prevent misunderstandings and foster a more inclusive work environment.

Conclusion

Effective team communication is a cornerstone of successful chiropractic practice. By fostering an environment of openness, practicing active listening, and addressing conflicts constructively, chiropractic teams can work more efficiently, enhance patient care, and create a positive workplace culture.

13.3 Conflict Resolution Strategies

Conflict in the workplace is inevitable, but effectively managing and resolving these conflicts is crucial for maintaining a positive work environment, especially in a chiropractic setting. Effective conflict resolution strategies can help prevent disagreements from escalating and ensure that the team remains focused on providing the best care to patients.

Identify the Root Cause

Begin by identifying the root cause of the conflict. Understanding the underlying issues, whether they stem from miscommunication, personality clashes, or differing work styles, is essential for finding a resolution that addresses the core problem.

Encourage Open Communication

Create an environment where team members feel safe expressing their thoughts and feelings without fear of reprisal. Encourage open communication and active listening, where each party is given the opportunity to share their perspective on the conflict.

Stay Neutral and Objective

When mediating conflicts, it's important to remain neutral and objective. Avoid taking sides or allowing personal biases to influence the resolution process. Focus on the facts and how the conflict impacts team dynamics and patient care.

Focus on Interests, Not Positions

Encourage team members to move beyond their initial positions or demands and explore their underlying interests. Understanding each party's needs and concerns can lead to more creative and mutually satisfactory solutions.

Seek Common Ground

Look for areas of agreement or common ground that can serve as a foundation for resolving the conflict. Highlighting shared goals, such as the well-being of patients or the success of the clinic, can help reorient the conversation towards collaboration.

Develop Win-Win Solutions

Aim for resolutions that are mutually beneficial to all parties involved. Win-win solutions that address the needs and interests of each party can lead to more lasting resolutions and strengthen team cohesion.

Implement and Follow Up

Once a resolution is agreed upon, implement the necessary changes or actions promptly. Follow up with all parties involved to ensure that the resolution is effective and that any lingering issues are addressed.

Promote a Culture of Respect

Fostering a workplace culture that values respect, diversity, and inclusivity can help prevent conflicts from arising in the first place. Regular team-building activities and training on communication and conflict resolution skills can also enhance team dynamics.

Use Mediation When Necessary

In cases where internal efforts to resolve the conflict are unsuccessful, consider using a neutral third-party mediator. Mediation can help facilitate discussions and lead to solutions that might not have been reached independently.

Conclusion

Effective conflict resolution is vital for maintaining a harmonious and productive work environment in a chiropractic setting. By employing these strategies, chiropractic practices can navigate conflicts constructively, preserving team relationships and ensuring that the focus remains on providing excellent patient care.

13.4 Exercise: 10 MCQs with Answers at the End

1. What is the first step in effectively resolving workplace conflicts?

A) Assigning blame

B) Identifying the root cause

C) Ignoring the issue

D) Increasing tension

2. Encouraging open communication in conflict resolution is important because it:

A) Wastes time

B) Allows each party to share their perspective

C) Creates more conflict

D) Discourages team involvement

3. Remaining neutral and objective during conflict resolution helps to:

A) Escalate the conflict

B) Influence the outcome with personal bias

C) Ensure fairness and impartiality

D) Show favoritism

4. Focusing on interests rather than positions encourages:

A) Stubbornness

B) Mutual understanding and compromise

C) Miscommunication

D) Competition

5. Finding common ground in a conflict involves:

A) Ignoring shared goals

B) Highlighting differences

C) Identifying shared objectives or agreements

D) Focusing on individual needs only

6. Win-win solutions in conflict resolution are characterized by:

A) Benefiting one party at the expense of another

B) Satisfying the needs of all parties involved

C) Leaving both parties unsatisfied

D) Avoiding the conflict altogether

7. The importance of follow-up after resolving a conflict is to:

A) Revisit the conflict

B) Ensure the resolution is effective and address any lingering issues

C) Blame participants

D) Ignore the outcome

8. Promoting a culture of respect in the workplace helps to:

A) Increase conflicts

B) Prevent conflicts from arising

C) Undermine team dynamics

D) Promote individualism over teamwork

9. Using a neutral third-party mediator is beneficial when:

   A) The conflict is easily resolved internally

   B) Internal efforts to resolve the conflict are unsuccessful

   C) Parties involved want to escalate the conflict

   D) There is no conflict

10. The ultimate goal of conflict resolution in a chiropractic setting is to:

   A) Focus on individual victories

   B) Maintain a harmonious and productive work environment

   C) Ignore team relationships

   D) Avoid addressing the issue

Answers:

1. B) Identifying the root cause

2. B) Allows each party to share their perspective

3. C) Ensure fairness and impartiality

4. B) Mutual understanding and compromise

5. C) Identifying shared objectives or agreements

6. B) Satisfying the needs of all parties involved

7. B) Ensure the resolution is effective and address any lingering issues

8. B) Prevent conflicts from arising

9. B) Internal efforts to resolve the conflict are unsuccessful

10. B) Maintain a harmonious and productive work environment

Chapter 14: Stress Management and Self-Care

14.1 Recognizing Signs of Burnout

Burnout is a state of emotional, physical, and mental exhaustion caused by excessive and prolonged stress. It occurs when one feels overwhelmed, emotionally drained, and unable to meet constant demands. Recognizing the signs of burnout is crucial for healthcare providers, including those in chiropractic practice, as it can significantly impact personal well-being and the quality of patient care.

Emotional Signs of Burnout:

- **Feeling drained or depleted of energy**

- **Increased feelings of cynicism or detachment from the job**

- **Sense of failure and self-doubt**

- **Feeling helpless, trapped, and defeated**

- **Decreased satisfaction and sense of accomplishment**

Physical Signs of Burnout:

- **Frequent illness due to lowered immune response**

- **Changes in appetite or sleep habits**

- Headaches, muscle pain, or gastrointestinal problems without a clear cause

Behavioral Signs of Burnout:

- Withdrawing from responsibilities

- Isolating oneself from others

- Procrastinating, taking longer to get things done

- Using food, drugs, or alcohol to cope

- Taking out frustrations on others

Work-related Signs of Burnout:

- Decreased productivity and effectiveness

- Feeling overwhelmed by work demands

- Difficulty concentrating and paying attention

- Lack of motivation and enthusiasm for work

- Avoiding work or calling in sick frequently

Recognizing the early signs of burnout is the first step in addressing and managing it. Effective strategies for managing burnout include seeking support, setting boundaries, practicing self-care, finding ways to reduce stress, and, if necessary, reevaluating one's professional path. For healthcare providers, maintaining personal well-being is not only essential for their health but is also critical to providing the best care for their patients.

Implementing regular self-assessments for burnout and encouraging an environment where staff feel comfortable discussing stress and burnout openly can help create a supportive workplace. Addressing burnout proactively can lead to healthier, more engaged, and more productive healthcare professionals.

14.2 Strategies for Personal Wellness

For individuals in the demanding field of chiropractic care, maintaining personal wellness is crucial. Balancing the pressures of patient care with personal health requires a comprehensive approach that encompasses physical, emotional, and mental well-being.

Physical Wellness Strategies:

- **Regular Exercise:** Engaging in regular physical activity can help reduce stress, improve mood, and enhance overall health. Activities such as yoga, swimming, or even brisk walking can be particularly effective.

- **Balanced Diet:** Eating a balanced diet rich in fruits, vegetables, whole grains, and lean proteins supports physical health and provides the energy needed for demanding days.

- **Adequate Rest:** Ensuring sufficient sleep each night is essential for recovery, cognitive function, and emotional stability.

Emotional Wellness Strategies:

- **Mindfulness and Meditation:** Practices like mindfulness and meditation can help manage stress, improve focus, and foster a sense of peace.

- **Hobbies and Interests:** Pursuing hobbies and interests outside of work can provide a much-needed escape, reduce stress, and increase life satisfaction.

- **Social Support:** Maintaining strong relationships with friends, family, and colleagues provides a support network that can offer comfort and assistance during challenging times.

Mental Wellness Strategies:

- **Setting Boundaries:** Learning to say no and setting clear boundaries between work and personal life can prevent overextension and burnout.

- **Time Management:** Effective time management techniques can help reduce work-related stress by ensuring tasks are prioritized and deadlines are met without overwhelming oneself.

- **Professional Help:** Seeking the assistance of a mental health professional when needed is a sign of strength and can provide strategies to cope with stress, anxiety, or depression.

Workplace Wellness Strategies:

- **Breaks During the Workday:** Taking short breaks throughout the day can help prevent fatigue and maintain high levels of concentration and patient care.

- **Ergonomic Workspaces:** Creating an ergonomic workspace can reduce the risk of physical strain and injury.

- **Continuing Education:** Engaging in continuing education not only advances professional knowledge but can also reinvigorate one's passion for their work.

Lifestyle Adjustments:

- **Digital Detox:** Periodically disconnecting from digital devices can reduce stress and improve quality of life.

- **Nature Time:** Spending time in nature has been shown to lower stress levels, improve mood, and enhance physical well-being.

- **Gratitude Practice:** Regularly practicing gratitude can shift focus from stressors to positive aspects of life, improving overall happiness.

Conclusion:

Implementing strategies for personal wellness allows chiropractic professionals to manage the stresses of their work while maintaining a high quality of life. By taking proactive steps towards physical, emotional, and mental health, individuals can ensure they are at their best for their patients and themselves.

14.3 Balancing Work and Personal Life

Achieving a balance between work and personal life is essential for the well-being of chiropractic professionals. The demanding nature of healthcare can often blur the lines between professional responsibilities and personal time, leading to stress, burnout, and a decline in the quality of care provided to patients. Here are strategies to help maintain this crucial balance.

Set Clear Boundaries:

Define clear boundaries between work and personal life. This may involve setting specific work hours, not taking work calls or emails at home, and having designated spaces for work and relaxation. Communicating these boundaries to colleagues, patients, and family members is also vital.

Prioritize Time Management:

Effective time management allows for dedicated time for both professional duties and personal activities. Utilize planning tools, such as calendars and to-do lists, to organize and prioritize tasks, ensuring that both work responsibilities and personal commitments are addressed.

Learn to Delegate:

Delegating tasks when possible can reduce workload and stress. Within the clinic, this might mean sharing responsibilities among staff members. At home, it might involve sharing household duties with family members or considering outside help.

Embrace Flexibility:

While structure is important, so is flexibility. Life is unpredictable, and the ability to adapt to changing circumstances while maintaining a sense of balance is crucial. This might mean adjusting work hours to accommodate a family event or taking a mental health day when needed.

Make Time for Self-care:

Regular self-care is non-negotiable for maintaining overall health and well-being. Activities such as exercise, hobbies, socializing, and relaxation should be integral parts of one's schedule, not afterthoughts.

Utilize Support Systems:

Relying on personal and professional support systems can provide relief and perspective. This includes family, friends, colleagues, and professional networks. Support groups or counseling services can also offer assistance and coping strategies.

Practice Mindfulness and Stress Reduction Techniques:

Incorporating mindfulness, meditation, or other stress reduction techniques into daily routines can help manage stress levels and improve emotional well-being, making it easier to navigate the demands of both work and personal life.

Take Vacations and Breaks:

Regular breaks, days off, and vacations are essential for rest and rejuvenation. Time away from work can help prevent burnout and renew one's enthusiasm and energy for their profession.

Evaluate and Adjust Regularly:

Life's demands change over time, so it's important to regularly evaluate and adjust the balance between work and personal life. This might involve reassessing priorities, changing work patterns, or finding new ways to manage stress.

Conclusion:

Balancing work and personal life in the chiropractic field requires intentional actions and strategies. By setting boundaries, managing time effectively, prioritizing self-care, and utilizing support systems, chiropractic professionals can maintain their well-being and continue to provide high-quality care to their patients.

14.4 Exercise: 10 MCQs with Answers at the End

1. What is a key strategy for balancing work and personal life?

   A) Ignoring personal needs

   B) Setting clear boundaries

   C) Working during vacations

   D) Taking work calls at all hours

2. Effective time management helps by:

   A) Increasing work hours

   B) Prioritizing tasks and dedicating time for personal activities

   C) Eliminating personal time

   D) Focusing solely on work tasks

3. The importance of delegating tasks is to:

   A) Increase individual workload

   B) Reduce stress and distribute workload

   C) Avoid responsibilities

   D) Complicate simple tasks

4. Flexibility in work-life balance is crucial for:

   A) Maintaining a rigid schedule

   B) Adapting to changing circumstances

   C) Ignoring personal commitments

   D) Decreasing productivity

5. Regular self-care is essential for:

   A) Decreasing well-being

   B) Increasing stress levels

   C) Maintaining overall health and well-being

   D) Isolating from social activities

6. Utilizing support systems can:

   A) Increase feelings of isolation

   B) Provide relief and perspective

   C) Discourage seeking help

   D) Promote independence from others

7. Mindfulness and stress reduction techniques aid in:

   A) Raising stress levels

   B) Managing stress and improving emotional well-being

   C) Ignoring work responsibilities

D) Decreasing focus and clarity

8. The purpose of taking vacations and breaks is to:

A) Avoid work responsibilities

B) Prevent burnout and renew enthusiasm for work

C) Isolate from colleagues

D) Reduce personal time

9. Regular evaluation and adjustment of work-life balance are necessary because:

A) Life's demands remain constant

B) Priorities and circumstances change over time

C) Work should always take precedence

D) Personal life is less important

10. A comprehensive approach to work-life balance includes:

A) Neglecting personal relationships

B) Focusing exclusively on professional development

C) Incorporating strategies for time management, self-care, and flexibility

D) Avoiding vacations and breaks to maximize work output

Answers:

1. B) Setting clear boundaries

2. B) Prioritizing tasks and dedicating time for personal activities

3. B) Reduce stress and distribute workload

4. B) Adapting to changing circumstances

5. C) Maintaining overall health and well-being

6. B) Provide relief and perspective

7. B) Managing stress and improving emotional well-being

8. B) Prevent burnout and renew enthusiasm for work

9. B) Priorities and circumstances change over time

10. C) Incorporating strategies for time management, self-care, and flexibility

Chapter 15: The Future of Chiropractic Care

15.1 Emerging Trends in Chiropractic Medicine

The field of chiropractic care is continually evolving, shaped by advancements in medical research, technology, and changing healthcare needs. Staying abreast of these trends is crucial for practitioners aiming to provide the best possible care to their patients. Here are some emerging trends in chiropractic medicine that are shaping the future of the profession.

Integration into Mainstream Healthcare

Chiropractic care is increasingly being integrated into mainstream healthcare settings, including hospitals and multidisciplinary clinics. This trend reflects a growing recognition of the value of chiropractic interventions in overall patient care, particularly for musculoskeletal conditions.

Focus on Evidence-based Practice

There is a growing emphasis on evidence-based practice within the chiropractic community. Research and clinical trials are expanding our understanding of the effectiveness of chiropractic treatments, leading to more informed care strategies and collaboration with other healthcare professionals.

Technological Advancements

Technology plays a significant role in the evolution of chiropractic care. Innovations such as digital imaging, electronic health records, and telehealth services are improving the efficiency of care delivery and patient management. Additionally, advanced treatment tools, including laser therapy and computer-assisted adjustment devices, are enhancing treatment precision and outcomes.

Patient-centered Care

The shift towards patient-centered care is influencing chiropractic practice. This approach emphasizes personalized care plans, patient education, and active patient involvement in health decisions. It fosters a holistic view of patient health, considering physical, emotional, and lifestyle factors.

Preventative and Wellness Care

Chiropractors are increasingly focusing on preventative care and overall wellness. Beyond treating existing conditions, practitioners are educating patients on healthy lifestyles, ergonomics, and preventative practices to support long-term health and prevent injuries.

Expansion of Telehealth Services

The use of telehealth in chiropractic care has surged, particularly in response to the COVID-19 pandemic. Telehealth services are making chiropractic care more accessible, allowing for consultations, follow-up appointments, and patient education to occur remotely.

Interdisciplinary Collaboration

Collaboration between chiropractors and professionals from other healthcare disciplines is becoming more common. This interdisciplinary approach enables comprehensive care plans that address various aspects of patient health, leading to better health outcomes.

Increased Focus on Nutrition and Lifestyle

Nutrition and lifestyle modifications are becoming integral parts of chiropractic care. Chiropractors are providing guidance on diet, exercise, and stress management to support the body's natural healing processes and promote overall wellness.

Regulatory and Educational Advances

Advancements in regulatory standards and chiropractic education are ensuring high levels of practice and professionalism. Continuing education requirements and standardized licensing examinations are elevating the quality of care provided by chiropractors.

Conclusion:

The future of chiropractic care is promising, driven by integration into mainstream healthcare, technological advancements, and a focus on evidence-based, patient-centered care. By embracing these emerging trends, chiropractors can continue to play a vital role in improving patient health and well-being.

15.2 The Evolving Role of Chiropractic Assistants

As the field of chiropractic care expands and adapts to new trends and technologies, the role of chiropractic assistants is also evolving. These vital team members are finding their responsibilities and opportunities for professional growth expanding in exciting ways.

Expanded Scope of Responsibilities

Chiropractic assistants are taking on more diverse roles within practices, beyond traditional administrative tasks. They are increasingly involved in patient education, managing telehealth services, and assisting with therapeutic treatments under the guidance of a chiropractor. This broadened scope requires a versatile skill set and a deep understanding of chiropractic care principles.

Increased Focus on Patient Experience

With the shift toward patient-centered care, chiropractic assistants play a crucial role in enhancing the patient experience. This includes everything from the first point of contact, ensuring comfortable and welcoming environments, to providing educational materials and follow-up care instructions. As such, interpersonal skills and empathy are more important than ever.

Integration of Technology

As chiropractic practices integrate more technology, assistants are often at the forefront of implementing and managing these systems. Proficiency with electronic health records (EHR), digital appointment scheduling, and telehealth platforms is becoming essential. Chiropractic assistants may also be involved in managing social media and online patient engagement strategies.

Participation in Wellness and Preventative Care

With the increasing emphasis on wellness and preventative care in chiropractic practices, assistants are becoming involved in delivering holistic health education. This might include advice on nutrition, exercise, and stress management, tailored to support the treatment plans developed by chiropractors.

Professional Development Opportunities

The evolving role of chiropractic assistants is accompanied by increased opportunities for professional development. There is a growing number of training programs and certifications available, covering areas such as office management, chiropractic therapy techniques, and health coaching. These opportunities not only enhance the capabilities of assistants but also the quality of care offered to patients.

Interdisciplinary Collaboration

As chiropractic care becomes more integrated with other healthcare services, assistants may find themselves coordinating care with other healthcare providers. This involves managing referrals, sharing patient information (with appropriate consent), and participating in team-based approaches to patient care.

Regulatory Compliance and Practice Management

Chiropractic assistants are increasingly involved in ensuring that practices comply with healthcare regulations, including patient privacy laws and occupational health and safety standards. They may also take on roles in practice management, including budgeting, inventory control, and staff training.

Conclusion:

The role of chiropractic assistants is becoming more dynamic and integral to the success of chiropractic practices. By embracing new responsibilities, engaging in continuous learning, and adapting to the needs of patients and practices, chiropractic assistants can significantly contribute to the evolving landscape of chiropractic care.

15.3 Preparing for the Future of Healthcare

As the healthcare landscape continues to evolve with technological advancements, demographic shifts, and changing patient expectations, it's crucial for chiropractic professionals, including chiropractors and their assistants, to prepare for the future. Adapting to these changes will ensure they continue to provide high-quality care and remain relevant in the healthcare ecosystem.

Embrace Technological Innovations

Staying abreast of technological advancements such as telehealth platforms, wearable health devices, and data analytics tools is essential. These technologies can enhance patient care, improve health outcomes, and streamline clinic operations. Continuous learning and training in new technologies will be key.

Focus on Integrated Care

The trend towards integrated care, where chiropractic services are part of a multidisciplinary approach to health, is expected to grow. Building strong collaborative relationships with other healthcare providers and understanding the broader healthcare system will be important for chiropractic professionals.

Enhance Skills in Patient-Centered Care

As patient expectations evolve, the ability to provide personalized, patient-centered care becomes increasingly important. This includes developing strong communication skills, understanding the social and environmental factors affecting health, and using shared decision-making processes.

Understand Healthcare Policy and Regulation Changes

Keeping informed about changes in healthcare policy and regulation that affect chiropractic practice is crucial. This knowledge will help practices navigate legal requirements, insurance coverage issues, and other administrative aspects of care delivery.

Prioritize Preventative and Holistic Care

With a growing emphasis on preventative care and wellness, chiropractic professionals are well-positioned to meet these needs. Expanding services to include wellness coaching, nutritional advice, and lifestyle modification support can address the holistic health needs of patients.

Develop Business and Management Skills

For those in or aspiring to leadership roles, developing business and management skills will be important for navigating the future healthcare landscape. This includes understanding healthcare economics, marketing, and strategic planning.

Commit to Lifelong Learning

The pace of change in healthcare means that lifelong learning is no longer optional but a necessity. Engaging in continuing education, attending professional conferences, and participating in professional networks can help chiropractic professionals stay current and adapt to future changes.

Promote Research and Evidence-Based Practice

Contributing to and staying informed about research in chiropractic care and related fields will support the integration of evidence-based practices into clinical care. This not only improves patient outcomes but also strengthens the profession's credibility within the healthcare community.

Conclusion:

Preparing for the future of healthcare requires chiropractic professionals to be proactive, flexible, and committed to continuous improvement. By embracing new technologies, integrating care, focusing on patient-centered services, and committing to lifelong learning, chiropractic professionals can navigate the changing healthcare landscape successfully and continue to make meaningful contributions to patient health and well-being.

15.4 Exercise: 10 MCQs with Answers at the End

1. What is crucial for chiropractic professionals to stay relevant in the evolving healthcare landscape?

    A) Ignoring technological advancements

    B) Avoiding interdisciplinary collaboration

    C) Embracing technological innovations

    D) Focusing solely on traditional practices

2. The trend towards what type of care is expected to grow in the future of healthcare?

    A) Isolated care

    B) Integrated care

    C) Outdated care methods

    D) Non-collaborative care

3. What type of care becomes increasingly important as patient expectations evolve?

    A) Impersonal care

    B) Patient-centered care

    C) Inflexible care

    D) Generic care

4. Why is it important to understand healthcare policy and regulation changes?

   A) To reduce clinic efficiency

   B) To navigate legal and administrative aspects of care delivery

   C) To complicate billing processes

   D) To ignore patient privacy concerns

5. What should chiropractic professionals expand their services to include, given the emphasis on preventative care?

   A) Only traditional chiropractic adjustments

   B) Wellness coaching and nutritional advice

   C) Less patient education

   D) Narrowing the scope of practice

6. Which skill set is important for those in leadership roles within chiropractic practices?

   A) Avoiding management responsibilities

   B) Business and management skills

   C) Refusing to adapt to changes

   D) Ignoring financial management

7. Continuous learning and training in new technologies are key for:

A) Decreasing patient care quality

B) Keeping abreast of technological advancements

C) Maintaining outdated treatment methods

D) Reducing practice efficiency

8. Engaging in what is no longer optional but a necessity for chiropractic professionals?

A) Lifelong learning

B) Avoiding professional development

C) Ignoring new research

D) Staying isolated from professional networks

9. What supports the integration of evidence-based practices into clinical care?

A) Disregarding current research

B) Promoting research and evidence-based practice

C) Sole reliance on anecdotal evidence

D) Avoiding updates to clinical guidelines

10. What can help chiropractic professionals navigate the changing healthcare landscape successfully?

   A) Resisting change at all costs

   B) Ignoring patient feedback

   C) Committing to continuous improvement

   D) Decreasing service quality

Answers:

1. C) Embracing technological innovations

2. B) Integrated care

3. B) Patient-centered care

4. B) To navigate legal and administrative aspects of care delivery

5. B) Wellness coaching and nutritional advice

6. B) Business and management skills

7. B) Keeping abreast of technological advancements

8. A) Lifelong learning

9. B) Promoting research and evidence-based practice

10. C) Committing to continuous improvement

Conclusion

As we've explored the multifaceted aspects of chiropractic practice, from patient care and office management to the future of healthcare, it's clear that the field is both challenging and rewarding. The chapters covered have provided insights into effective patient communication, inventory management, safety protocols, financial management, and the importance of leadership and teamwork. Additionally, we've delved into stress management, the evolving role of chiropractic assistants, and preparing for the future of healthcare.

Key takeaways include the importance of embracing technological innovations, fostering a patient-centered approach, prioritizing continuous professional development, and maintaining a balance between work and personal life. Moreover, the significance of adopting evidence-based practices, engaging in interdisciplinary collaboration, and staying adaptable to the changing healthcare landscape has been emphasized.

For chiropractic professionals and assistants, the journey is one of lifelong learning and adaptation, with the ultimate goal of enhancing patient health and well-being. By committing to excellence, embracing growth opportunities, and navigating the challenges with resilience and integrity, chiropractic practitioners can continue to make a significant impact on the healthcare field.

The exploration of these topics serves as a foundation for building a successful, fulfilling career in chiropractic care and contributing to the broader healthcare community. With dedication and passion, chiropractic professionals can look forward to a future where they continue to improve lives, one adjustment at a time.

*The best way to thank an author is
to
write a review.*